Second Edition

Moral Issues in Health Care

AN INTRODUCTION TO MEDICAL ETHICS

Terrance McConnell

University of North Carolina at Greensboro

Wadsworth Publishing Company
I⟨T⟩P® An International Thomson Publishing Company

Belmont, CA • Albany, NY • Bonn • Boston • Cincinnati • Detroit •
Johannesburg • London • Madrid • Melbourne • Mexico City • New York •
Paris • San Francisco • Singapore • Tokyo • Toronto • Washington

Philosophy Editor: *Peter Adams*
Editorial Assistant: *Greg Brueck*
Marketing Manager: *Dave Garrison*
Project Editor: *Jerilyn Emori*
Print Buyer: *Barbara Britton*
Permissions Editor: *Robert Kauser*

Advertising Project Manager: *Joseph Jodar*
Designer: *Wendy LaChance*
Copy Editor: *Laura Larson*
Cover Designer: *Madeleine Budnick*
Compositor: *Scratchgravel Publishing Services*
Printer: *Malloy Lithographing, Inc.*

Printed in the United States of America
1 2 3 4 5 6 7 8 9 10

For more information, contact Wadsworth Publishing Company, 10 Davis Drive, Belmont, CA 94002,
or electronically at http://www.thomson.com/wadsworth.html

International Thomson Publishing Europe
Berkshire House 168-173
High Holborn
London, WC1V 7AA, England

International Thomson Editores
Campos Eliseos 385, Piso 7
Col. Polanco
11560 México D.F. México

Thomas Nelson Australia
102 Dodds Street
South Melbourne 3205
Victoria, Australia

International Thomson Publishing Asia
221 Henderson Road
#05-10 Henderson Building
Singapore 0315

Nelson Canada
1120 Birchmount Road
Scarborough, Ontario
Canada M1K 5G4

International Thomson Publishing Japan
Hirakawacho Kyowa Building, 3F
2-2-1 Hirakawacho
Chiyoda-ku, Tokyo 102, Japan

International Thomson Publishing GmbH
Königswinterer Strasse 418
53227 Bonn, Germany

International Thomson Publishing Southern Africa
Building 18, Constantia Park
240 Old Pretoria Road
Halfway House, 1685 South Africa

Library of Congress Cataloging-in-Publication Data
McConnell, Terrance C.
    Moral issues in health care : an introduction to medical ethics /
Terrance McConnell. — 2nd ed.
        p.   cm.
    Includes index.
    ISBN 0-534-24744-X
    1. Medical ethics.   I. Title.
R724.M292   1996
174'.2—dc20   96-19413

*This book is printed on
acid-free recycled paper.*

Contents

PREFACE

ANYONE TEACHING A COURSE in biomedical ethics has a number of decisions to make. The first concerns a selection of books. Many are available; most are anthologies, not single-authored texts. My own experience suggests that there are advantages and disadvantages associated with each. Anthologies typically present instructors with a richer array of topics from which to choose and many different authors representing multiple points of view. These are significant advantages. The main difficulty that I have encountered is that the articles collected in anthologies have normally been published in scholarly journals, and so they often address narrow issues and have been written for professional readers. Although this type of presentation can offer students an exhilarating challenge, it can also create frustrations.

The main disadvantage of single-authored texts is that the author's biases may creep in; it is difficult to present all points of view objectively. The advantages, however, are that the author can aim for a more general audience, provide an overview of the various issues, and explain the strengths and weaknesses of the competing positions. My goal in this text is to explain the most fundamental moral principles and their role in particular moral problems that arise in medical contexts. I strive to provide a general framework in which readers can place and examine numerous moral questions. I do not attempt to provide guidance regarding very specific problems; here, individual judgment is required.

Another decision that must be made concerns what issues to address. Most readers know that there are enough issues in biomedical ethics to teach several courses without duplication. I have, of necessity, omitted many topics, and I do not mean to suggest that they are unimportant. My choice of issues is the result of my teaching biomedical ethics (seventeen years) and serving on an ethics committee at a local hospital (five years and counting). Over the years, I have tried different topics, and the ones covered here are those in which my students have shown the most interest. In some cases, I have been surprised (for example, the enthusiastic response to issues concerning the use of human subjects in experiments, the discussion of public policies for obtaining scarce medical resources); in other cases, the reaction was more predictable (for example, abortion, euthanasia). I will explain very briefly the topics I have included.

Chapter 1 deals with certain issues in ethical theory. The bulk of this chapter explores the rather theoretical issue of whether ethical judgments are merely subjective (simply a matter of individual taste) or are objective (open to reasoned examination). In this discussion, at times the going is tedious and some readers will be annoyed. But my own past experience has indicated that it is important to face this issue directly and immediately; it will arise at some point. This chapter also explains some basic moral principles and some broad ethical theories. These explanations are rather brief; my strategy is to state the principles and then explore them further as they arise in the discussion of specific moral problems. This approach has worked well for me in the classroom.

Chapter 2 begins by explaining several models of the health care practitioner–patient relationship, models that differ on how decision making in medicine should be made. Explaining these models requires invoking some of the basic principles mentioned in Chapter 1. In addition, two specific issues are addressed here. One concerns confidentiality. The goals in this discussion are first to explain why confidentiality in medicine is morally important, and then to ask whether there are any circumstances in which health care professionals are justified in breaching a patient's confidence. The other issue concerns being truthful with patients. Here the goals are first to explain the moral bases for being honest with patients about their diagnoses and prognoses, and then to ask whether it is ever morally justified to withhold the truth from a patient. I do not try to settle the issues once and for all; instead, I try to present the strongest cases I can for confidentiality and honesty, and then indicate what some of the hard cases are for these positions.

Chapter 3 concerns the topic of informed consent. One main goal here is to explain, in terms of basic moral principles, why competent patients have the right to refuse recommended medical treatment. Another goal is to explain the moral limits on surrogates who might wish to refuse medical treatment for an incompetent. Yet another goal is to explain the elements that make up *informed* consent. Again, hard cases that challenge the orthodox views will be presented.

Chapter 4 addresses various issues surrounding euthanasia and the withdrawal of life-sustaining treatment. Here topics include distinguishing various types of euthanasia, the pros and cons of legalizing euthanasia, physician-assisted suicide, and the basic principles for guiding surrogates in deciding whether to withdraw or withhold life-sustaining treatment from an incompetent patient. Some of the classic cases in medical ethics will be used here as illustrations.

Chapter 5 concerns the controversial issue of abortion. In many ways, this chapter was the most difficult to write. Here the goal is to explain representative positions from the whole spectrum on this issue and to explain the main criticisms of those positions. I have tried to be as objective as possible in this presentation.

Chapter 6 addresses an array of issues that arise when human subjects are used in medical research. Again, the basic principles introduced in Chapter 1 are employed to explain the issues. Two important topics are whether it is ever permissible to use subjects without their fully informed consent and whether it is ever permissible to conduct research in which subjects are placed at risk. Classic cases from the recent history of medical research are used as illustrations.

Chapter 7 deals with two issues that arise because medical resources are sometimes scarce. One issue concerns allocation. If the demand for a medical resource exceeds the supply, only some in need will benefit. Selecting who will receive that resource is a very difficult moral issue. Various accounts of how such decisions should be made will be examined. The other issue concerns acquisition. If a valuable resource is in short supply, then society needs to ask whether steps can be taken to increase the supply. Here, then, we will examine different policies that society might adopt for obtaining scarce medical resources (such as organs for transplantation) and the moral implications of those policies.

One obvious omission deserves an explanation. I do not in this edition have a chapter on the right to health care. A major reason for this is concern about the length of this book; another chapter would make it too long. Another reason is my judgment that this topic is so complex and so rapidly changing that anything short of a book-length treatment of it is apt to be inadequate. Fortunately, publishers now enable instructors to order portions of books for their courses, and so this text could be easily supplemented with essays on the right to health care from another work.

What I do here is present an outline or overview of some basic issues in biomedical ethics. While I attempt to provide a framework, in no way do I suppose that what I say is the final word. All of these topics are ones on which there is ongoing debate. Any author would be arrogant to suppose that he or she has settled the matters, once and for all. When I teach, I sometimes urge my students to regard the entire experience as a dialogue whose participants are the instructor, the author or authors of their books, and the class members themselves. I invite readers to view this book in the same way.

Approximately 50 percent of the students to whom I have taught medical ethics over the last decade and a half have been enrolled in our university's nursing and pre-med programs. The other 50 percent have come from various disciplines. I have learned from many of these students. Their reactions make clear what topics I am presenting well and what ones I am explaining poorly. The students in medically related fields have been especially generous in sharing their experiences; much that I have learned from them is incorporated in this book.

When philosophers discuss any topic, obviously they have a tendency to be very theoretical. Just as obviously, any useful contribution to the field of biomedical ethics must have practical applications. In this regard, I have learned much from others. I especially want to thank three Greensboro physicians with whom I have discussed many cases and from whom I have learned much: Timothy Lane, Rita Layson, and Stewart Rogers. I have also been educated in many ways by fellow members of the Ethics Committee at the Moses H. Cone Memorial Hospital in Greensboro, North Carolina. Our case consultations have contributed enormously to my understanding of the issues discussed in this book. I also thank Greensboro attorney Kay Hagan for excellent help on matters regarding bioethics and the law. A three-year stint on the Institutional Review Board at the Moses Cone Hospital also gave me a better and more practical perspective on ethical issues in medical research.

Four different reviewers for Wadsworth provided comments and suggestions on earlier versions of this work. In most cases the comments were constructive, and in each case I learned something useful. While I did not always take the advice of these reviewers, I followed it often and I thank them for their suggestions: Robin S. Dillon, Lehigh University; Harvey Green, Tulane University; Edward Langerak, Saint Olaf College; and Pat Sheer, Phoenix College.

I thank the staff members of Wadsworth Publishing Company who worked with me on this project, especially philosophy editor Peter Adams and project editor Jerilyn Emori. Their support and guidance were very helpful. I also thank Laura Larson, my copy editor, whose work was outstanding; in many places, she helped me find ways to clarify the text, while always retaining the original meaning.

A special thanks is owed to my wife, Marilyn Lee McConnell, for her expert advice on medical matters and her encouragement.

CHAPTER 1

Ethical Theory

ETHICS IS THE STUDY of moral beliefs. After briefly indicating the various ways in which moral beliefs can be examined, this chapter will focus on whether moral disputes can be resolved rationally. Are there correct answers to moral questions, or is it possible that none of several disputants is mistaken? If there are correct answers to moral questions, it is important to examine theories that purport to provide these. In the latter portions of this chapter, several normative theories of particular interest in medical ethics will be discussed.

THE STUDY OF ETHICS

What does the study of ethics involve? Definitions of "ethics" given in textbooks are seldom helpful. You might read, for example, that ethics is the philosophical study of moral beliefs. Or you might be told that ethics involves reasoned discourse about morality. Such definitions, however, are not particularly helpful. The approach here is to distinguish three different ways to study moral beliefs and to indicate which will be pursued in this book.

The first way to study moral beliefs is called *descriptive ethics* and is concerned with stating the actual moral beliefs of some person or group of persons. This sort of inquiry may be engaged in by anthropologists, sociologists, and historians. The activity is an empirical one. The goal is to describe what certain people *think* or believe is right or wrong. In descriptive ethics, no evaluation of these beliefs takes place. If an instructor were to distribute a survey to members of the class asking about their views on abortion, euthanasia, and capital punishment, and then compile and report the results with no evaluative comments, this would be an example of descriptive ethics.

The second way to study moral beliefs is called *normative ethics*. Those engaged in this activity are concerned not merely with what someone thinks is right or wrong but with what *really* is right or wrong. The focus of normative ethics lies in the justification that can be given to support those beliefs. Issues of normative ethics arise at different levels of specificity. The most obvious instance of a question in normative ethics concerns the moral status of a particular act. A health care practitioner might ask, for example, whether lying to this patient in these particular circumstances is warranted. Or one might wonder whether breaching the confidence of this patient in this special situation is justified. At a higher level of generality, one might be concerned about the moral status of certain *types* of actions. A health care practitioner might ask whether lying to a patient is ever right or whether it is ever permissible to breach the confidence of a patient. These concerns are still in the area of normative ethics, but at a higher level of generality. At an even higher level of abstraction, one might wonder what, if anything, all right actions have in common or what all wrong actions have in common. If, for example, one has concluded that lying to patients is always wrong and that breaching the confidence of patients is always wrong, one might wonder what the common features are that make acts of these two types wrong.

Metaethics is the third way to study moral beliefs. This approach involves questions about the field of ethics itself. The metaethicist steps back and tries to analyze what is going on when people engage in normative ethics. The metaethicist might observe, for example, that when people discuss moral issues, they frequently use terms such as *right, wrong, good,* and *bad.* Analyzing the meanings of these common terms as they occur in moral discourse is an activity of metaethics. More generally, metaethics has as its goal to reveal and examine the presuppositions of normative ethics.

Our study of medical ethics will primarily be an exercise in normative ethics. We will be asking such questions as these: Should a physician or nurse always tell a dying patient the truth about his condition? Is it ever permissible for a health care practitioner to breach the confidence of her patient? And more importantly, we will examine the kinds of reasons or arguments that can be given to support particular answers to these questions. We will be interested in descriptive ethics only when we examine briefly the various codes of medical ethics, such as the Hippocratic Oath and the American Medical Association's Principles of Medical Ethics. The purpose of examining these codes will be to see what certain members of the medical community have thought about some of these issues.

SUBJECTIVISM AND OBJECTIVISM

Before embarking on this journey in normative ethics, we must address the most fundamental question raised in the area of metaethics. If we do not come to terms with this issue at the outset, the whole journey may seem pointless. The question concerns the very nature of moral judgments. When the metaethicist steps back and observes what is going on when people engage in normative discourse, one point is striking. People disagree about moral issues. Arguments are often heated, and sometimes the actions people take in the name of morality are even violent. One cannot help but wonder whether there are correct and incorrect answers to these questions or whether it is all just a matter of opinion. Two schools of thought—two metaethical theories—emerge here. We shall call these *objectivism* and *subjectivism*.

When a discipline or area of inquiry is *objective*, there are correct and incorrect answers to issues in that area. By contrast, when a discipline or area of inquiry is *subjective*, questions in that area do not have correct or incorrect answers. If an area is subjective, then assertions concerning that matter are just a matter of opinion or taste. An area that presumably most agree is subjective is taste in ice cream. If one person says that chocolate ice cream is good and another says that it is not good, we do not typically think that one is correct and the other is mistaken. Rather, we think that taste in ice cream is subjective. On the other hand, disciplines such as chemistry, physics, and history, where history is understood simply as reporting dates and facts, are widely thought to be objective. Thus, if two people disagree about the chemical makeup of a particular solution, one of them must be wrong. Similarly, if one person says that George Washington died in 1799 and another claims that he died in 1800, at least one of them is mistaken.

We can now define the terms *objective* and *subjective* more precisely. Moral judgments, such as "Act A is right (wrong)," are *objective* just in case for any two people, if one affirms the judgment "Act A is right" and the other denies it, at least one of them is mistaken. On the other hand, moral judgments such as "Act A is right" are *subjective* just in case it is possible for there to be two people such that one of them affirms the judgment "Act A is right" and the other denies it, and neither is mistaken. The subjectivist might analyze a debate about the morality of abortion, for example, as follows. One person, P1, thinks that abortion is always wrong; a second, P2, thinks that abortion in certain circumstances is permissible. Neither P1 nor P2 is incorrect. It is all a matter of opinion. The objectivist, by contrast, must say that the moral belief of at least one of these disputants is mistaken. The objectivist need not say that he *knows*, at the moment, which is mistaken, however. Whether there are answers and whether we know them are two different issues.

Three points about the definitions just offered should be noticed. First, these definitions can, with suitable alteration, be adapted to any discipline. Indeed, we can ask *meta*questions about chemistry, physics, mathematics, psychology, history, and any other discipline, and objectivism and subjectivism will emerge as competing metatheories regarding each discipline. Second, the plausibility of the proposed definitions is confirmed by the fact that they accord with the examples given earlier. Clearly the issue of whether chocolate ice cream is really good is one that most think is subjective; indeed, it seems that two people can disagree about such a matter and neither be mistaken. But if we are talking about the chemical makeup of a particular solution or the year in which George Washington died, if one person affirms a judgment about either and the other denies it, we think that at least one must be mistaken. Third, objectivism is defined with the qualification "*at least* one must be mistaken," because both (or all) disputants may be mistaken, depending on the nature of the dispute. To return to a previous example, if one person says that George Washington died in 1799 and another says that he died in 1800, it is possible that both are mistaken. On the other hand, if the second party simply denied that Washington died in 1799, then only one will be incorrect.

Many people claim to be subjectivists about ethics. But some reject objectivism for bad reasons, reasons that confuse objectivism with a related but different thesis called *absolutism*. According to absolutism, all moral rules hold without exception. Someone who says that the essence of morality consists in the Ten Commandments and that each commandment holds without exception is an absolutist. Or, someone might say that the usual prohibitions against killing, stealing, and breaking promises all hold without exception. Many people deny that moral judgments are objective because they reject absolutism; they think that there are legitimate exceptions to moral rules and that this belief commits them to subjectivism. This reasoning is specious, however, because one who holds that moral judgments are objective need not hold that moral absolutism is true. An objectivist is only committed to saying that one general moral principle holds without exception and that principle, whatever it might be, provides the basis for identifying the exceptions.

This point can be illustrated by explaining a notion that contrasts with absolutism, namely, *context dependence*. A moral judgment is context-dependent if the same kind of action can be right in one context or set of circumstances and wrong in a different context. Many people reject moral absolutism and instead accept the notion of context dependence. Many believe, for example, that though a person normally ought to tell the truth, it is permissible to lie to a would-be murderer concerning the whereabouts of his intended victim. And though most of us believe that a person normally ought to keep a promise, we think that breaking a promise to meet a friend for lunch is permissible to save the life of an accident victim.

It seems plausible, then, to hold that moral judgments are context-dependent. But the objectivist can allow this; the objectivist need not be an absolutist. The objectivist can allow that exceptions to moral rules are possible, as long as those exceptions can be identified in a principled way. This is best illustrated by first noting the relationship between a general moral principle and particular moral rules. For purposes of illustration, consider the following general moral principle: "Always do that which will promote the general welfare." The following diagram shows some of the particular moral rules that might follow from this general principle:

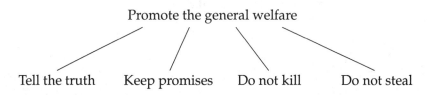

In most cases, a person will have to live by these rules to promote the general welfare; that is, normally abiding by these rules will better promote the general welfare than violating the rules. But in certain extreme circumstances, an agent may have to break some of these rules to promote better the general welfare. Cases mentioned in the previous paragraph indicate situations in which the general welfare is better promoted by not telling the truth and by breaking a promise. Similarly, killing a person intent on mayhem may be necessary to promote the general welfare, assuming that no less forceful means is available to stop this person. And one can imagine situations in which people must steal to feed their families.

So, though these rules hold for the most part, there are exceptions to them. What is important to realize here is that these exceptions are not determined by arbitrary whim; they are made on a principled basis. Given the general principle, if an instructor's being truthful with her class is what best promotes the general welfare, that is what she ought to do; and if lying to the would-be murderer best promotes the general welfare, that is what she ought to do. It is compatible with objectivism to allow for exceptions to moral rules that are determined on a principled basis.

If the principle "Promote the general welfare" is correct, then in each situation what one really ought to do is that action among the alternatives available that best promotes the general welfare. In one situation, an action of a certain type may best promote the general welfare; in another situation, it may not. This condition is context dependent, and the objectivist can allow for this. And, it is important to note, different principles from the one mentioned can accommodate context dependence. Note that if one's principle were "Obey God's commands," the same sort of considerations emerges, assuming that God issues commands to agents in particular situations. Note, too, that though objectivists need not be absolutists, absolutists must be objectivists; for the absolutist certainly holds that there are correct and incorrect answers to moral questions. Absolutism represents only one species of objectivism.

Arguments for Subjectivism: A Critical Assessment

If someone's reason for affirming subjectivism is based on a rejection of absolutism, these grounds are insufficient. For objectivists too can reject absolutism. Other reasons, however, have been given in support of subjectivism. A critical examination of these will follow.

An *argument* is a chain of reasoning consisting of statements, called *premises*, the affirmation of which is designed to convince others to accept yet another statement, called the *conclusion*. An attorney, for example, presents arguments to members of the jury trying to convince them of her client's innocence. Here we are interested in arguments that have been given in support of subjectivism. In ordinary conversation, arguments are not usually stated fully; premises are typically understood or assumed but left unstated. Philosophers call such a pattern of reasoning an *enthymeme*, an argument with one or more suppressed premises. Arguments for subjectivism are typically presented as reasons in an enthymematic form. In examining these, we shall first state the reason, and then show its full form, including the suppressed premises. Only by doing this can we adequately assess the argument.

The first reason given to support subjectivism is that there is widespread disagreement about moral matters, both between and within societies. Furthermore, people rarely change their minds about moral matters. In converting this reason to a full-fledged argument, we will learn something about the nature of reasons. Reasons are universal in the following sense. Suppose I say that Pedro is tall. You ask why I think that. I say, "Because he is over six feet in height." If that is really why I think that Pedro is tall, then I must say that anyone over six feet in height is tall; otherwise I am either being inconsistent or not stating my real reason fully. Thus, if the reason that someone offers for holding that ethics is subjective is that there is widespread disagreement in the field of ethics, then that person must grant that the presence of widespread disagreement alone shows that any discipline is subjective. The argument underlying this first reason, then, has two premises. The first is general, and the second is more specific. They may be stated as follows:

1a. **Whenever there is widespread disagreement in an area (discipline), that area is subjective.**
1b. **There is widespread disagreement about moral matters.**
1c. **Therefore, morality is subjective.**

For an argument to be convincing, two things must obtain. First, the reasoning must be correct. That is, the relationship between the premises and the conclusion must be such that *if* the premises are true, then the conclusion must also be true; one cannot, without inconsistency, affirm the truth of the premises and deny the truth of the conclusion. Second, the premises must be true.

Without pretending to give a course in logic, it should be clear that the *pattern of reasoning* in the first argument is correct. *If* premises 1a and 1b are true, one must accept the conclusion, 1c. So to assess this argument, we must ask whether the premises are true. We may grant, for the sake of argument, that premise 1b is true. In our own society we can observe serious disagreement among people regarding such issues as abortion, euthanasia, and capital punishment. And it seems that anthropologists and sociologists have provided ample evidence of disagreement between various societies. We should not exaggerate these differences, however; for every society seems in some way to affirm the importance of norms prohibiting killing, stealing, and dishonesty.

Our focus, however, should be on premise 1a. This premise seems doubtful. The mere fact that there is widespread disagreement in an area does not show that that area is subjective. Just because people have arrived at conflicting answers about an issue, it does not follow that there is no correct answer to that matter. Notice that there is not universal agreement in the various sciences, but few draw the inference that these areas are subjective. Physicists, chemists, and biologists disagree among themselves about many basic issues. At one time in the history of science, astronomers could not agree whether the sun or the earth is the center of our universe. And though many people believe that diseases are caused by viruses, some think that they are caused by demons or gods. These considerations tempt few to conclude that what the center of our universe is and what the cause of disease is are merely matters of opinion. Or consider an even simpler example. Suppose that there are four eye witnesses to a crime. Testimony from each is solicited about the perpetrator's height, weight, clothing, and the like. In all likelihood, the reports of these eye witnesses will differ on many points about the details. But that disagreement does not mean that what the height, weight, and attire of the perpetrator were is a subjective matter. All of this shows that more than widespread disagreement is needed to establish subjectivism. Thus, premise 1a is false and the first argument for subjectivism should be rejected.

The second reason to support subjectivism is that people acquire their moral beliefs from their parents, peer groups, and their particular society. The moral beliefs people have depend in large part on the environment in which they have been raised. Moral beliefs are not discovered; it is rather a matter of assimilation. Moreover, since people have different environments, agreement about moral matters may never be achieved. Again, this reason is stated in an abbreviated form, and the full-fledged argument underlying it is this:

2a. **Whenever beliefs in an area are acquired from others and not discovered, that area is subjective.**

2b. **Moral beliefs are acquired from others, not discovered.**

2c. **Therefore, morality is subjective.**

Like the previous argument, the pattern of reasoning here is correct, and so whether one should accept the conclusion, 2c, depends on whether the premises, 2a and 2b, are true. Let us grant the truth of 2b and focus on 2a. This premise seems doubtful. How someone acquires a belief seems irrelevant to the assessment of that belief. For example, how Darwin arrived at his theory of evolution does not affect our assessment of that theory. Similarly, then, how someone acquires moral beliefs is not relevant to the correctness/incorrectness of those beliefs. It should be noted, too, that people acquire almost all of their beliefs from others—beliefs about science and history, as well as morality. So if the reasoning in this second argument shows that morality is subjective, it would also show that areas such as the sciences and history are subjective, and this is a position that few are willing to adopt.

A third reason in support of subjectivism appeals to the uncertainty of our moral judgments. Moral judgments are very complicated, and we can never be certain of their accuracy. Numerous examples might be cited to illustrate this point. A woman may have good medical reasons for aborting the fetus she is carrying, but her religious beliefs may be such that she has qualms about doing so. She may think that both sets of considerations are pertinent, but she does not know how to resolve the conflict. If the uncertainty of our judgments alone shows that morality is subjective, then any other field that is complicated will be one that proponents of this argument must hold is subjective. The full argument can thus be stated:

3a. **Whenever judgments in an area are complicated or uncertain, that area is subjective.**

3b. **Judgments in morality are complicated and uncertain.**

3c. **Therefore, morality is uncertain.**

The pattern or form of reasoning in this argument is the same as the previous two, and so we shall not challenge that. But again we must examine the plausibility of the two premises. We may grant the truth of premise 3b; it is hard to deny that at least some moral judgments are very complicated, and our uncertainty is quite warranted. But two points count against this argument. First, this argument is not really for subjectivism. Instead, it is an argument for moral skepticism, the view that we do not have genuine knowledge about morality, and as a result all of our judgments in that area are uncertain. Subjectivism is the view that there are no correct/incorrect answers to moral questions; skepticism is simply the view that we do not know what the answers are. These are two very different positions. Second, premise 3a seems dubious. Many other fields are complicated and the judgments in those areas are uncertain, but few conclude that they are subjective. Certainly this is true of the various sciences, and it is also true of historical claims. Consider how difficult it is to be certain about statements concerning the distant past. There are, then, good reasons to reject this third argument.

A fourth reason in support of subjectivism claims that there are no moral authorities, no moral experts.[1] Some have even suggested that the very notion of moral expertise is an absurdity. This idea is expressed when people ask, "Who are you to say what is right?" This reason gains additional credibility when the presence of experts in other areas—areas believed to be objective—is noted. For example, there are experts in the various branches of the physical sciences. So if morality were objective, there should be moral experts, too. The full argument implicit in this reason may be stated as follows:

4a. If there are no experts or authorities in an area, that area is subjective.

4b. There are no moral experts.

4c. Therefore, morality is subjective.

Again, the pattern of reasoning underlying this argument is correct; *if* the premises are true, the conclusion must also be true. But are the premises true? There are several criticisms designed to show that they are not true.

First, premise 4a seems doubtful. There is a distinction, obscured by 4a, between whether there are answers to a given question and whether anyone knows those answers. Objectivists in ethics are only committed to saying that there are correct answers regarding what agents ought to do in particular circumstances; they need not say that anyone knows those answers. Of course, since there are experts in other areas believed to be objective, objectivists owe us an explanation as to why there are no moral experts. But explanations are available. Objectivists might say, for example, that ethics is a very difficult field; there is still no established body of knowledge in the area of morality, and thus there are no experts.

Few, however, will be satisfied with this first critical response as it stands. People have been grappling with moral questions for several thousand years. As a result, it is reasonable to expect that some progress will have been made and that a body of knowledge will have developed. So even though this first critical response is correct as far as it goes, more is needed.

A second response to the "no moral experts" argument challenges the adequacy of premise 4b. Objectivists can claim that there are in fact moral experts. Making such a claim, however, invites two other questions: Who are these alleged moral experts? And why is there such a widespread opinion that there are no such experts?

To say that there are moral experts initially sounds arrogant, but that interpretation is due to inappropriate connotations surrounding the word *expert*. An expert is not someone who is infallible or omniscient; rather, an expert is someone who knows more about a given area or subject matter than most others. Experts in all fields make mistakes. A moral expert may simply be someone who has read, written, and thought more about moral issues than most of the general population. It should not be surprising if someone has spent time deliberating about moral issues that such a person will be better able than most to articulate general moral principles, explain their rationale, show how they are interrelated, and anticipate conflicts among them. Persons who may qualify as moral experts in this sense include moral philosophers, certain theologians, and some counselors. Once the notion of an expert is made sufficiently modest, denying premise 4b should not seem so outrageous.

But why do so many doubt that there are moral experts? One reason may be this. If a person has a problem in an area widely believed to be objective—say, one of the physical sciences—and goes to an expert in that area for advice, that person is likely to receive straightforward, unequivocal advice. But, a defender of premise 4b will retort, if one goes to an alleged moral expert with a difficult problem, one seldom receives a straightforward answer. Instead, one is likely to receive a reply qualified with "ifs," "buts," and the like. And that response fosters the suspicion that there are no moral experts after all. The critic of premise 4b—that is, the defender of moral expertise—can rebut this challenge, however.

Two points are relevant. First, it is not true that recognized experts in other fields always give unequivocal advice. Physicians are experts about medical matters, but they often give highly qualified advice; in so doing, they are acknowledging the difficulty of their field and their own fallibility. Similarly, those who go to attorneys for legal advice do not always receive straightforward recommendations. Again, the expert in question may recognize that because of the difficulty of the issue, she is not warranted in giving an oversimplified response.

Second, objectivists can explain why moral experts are not typically positioned to give unequivocal advice (without denying that there are correct answers to moral issues). To know what one ought to do in a particular situation, one needs knowledge of two sorts: (1) knowledge of the applicable general moral principle and (2) knowledge of the facts of that particular situation to which the principle applies. Moral experts will have the former knowledge, of course, but there is no reason to believe that they will have expertise regarding the latter. Consider this example. Suppose, just for the sake of illustration, that the following moral principle is plausible: if the chances of severe genetic deformity are great, a couple should not have children. Now suppose that you and your spouse go to a moral expert and ask that person whether it is permissible for you to have children. For her to answer this question, she needs to know the applicable moral principle; but she also must be knowledgeable about genetics in general and the genetic history of you and your spouse in particular. Without all of this information, an unqualified answer to your question would be irresponsible. And it is unlikely that anyone will have all of this knowledge at her fingertips, which is one reason that medical ethics is an interdisciplinary field. It requires knowledge from many areas, and no one person is likely to have all of that knowledge.

The fifth reason in support of subjectivism is perhaps the most popular. It holds that subjectivism is superior to objectivism because of the moral consequences of those two views. More specifically, it claims that objectivism leads to dogmatism (the unwillingness to listen to criticisms of one's own views) and intolerance (imposing one's views on others), while subjectivism leads to open-mindedness and tolerance. Since the latter are preferable to the former, subjectivism is the more plausible view. The full argument lying behind this reason may be stated as follows:

5a. **Whenever the consequences of a view are implausible, that view itself is implausible.**

5b. **The consequences of objectivism are implausible because it leads to dogmatism and intolerance, while subjectivism avoids these undesirable consequences.**

5c. **Therefore, objectivism is implausible, and subjectivism is preferable.**

Again, the structure of the underlying reasoning here is correct. But are the premises true? We may grant the plausibility of the major premise, 5a. But premise 5b is another matter; it can be shown to be false, for several reasons. First, neither open-mindedness nor tolerance follows from subjectivism. To be open-minded is to be willing to change one's moral views in light of the criticisms of others. But subjectivists have no reason to alter their moral views because of criticisms. According to subjectivism, ultimately one's moral judgments are neither correct nor incorrect. So subjectivists cannot take others' criticisms seriously, for those criticisms cannot show that the subjectivists' opinions are mistaken. And why should subjectivists be tolerant of the moral opinions of others? Nothing in subjectivism suggests an obligation not to impose one's views on another. Subjectivism holds that morality is a matter of taste, and if one has a taste for intolerance nothing in subjectivism can denounce this.

Second, if it follows from subjectivism that moral agents ought to be open-minded and tolerant, then subjectivism would be self-refuting. For if a moral agent *ought* to be tolerant or *ought* to be open-minded, then at least one moral judgment is correct and the opposing judgment is incorrect, which is contrary to subjectivism.

Finally, objectivists need be neither dogmatic nor intolerant. Objectivists say that there are right and wrong answers to moral questions, not that they know what those answers are. Moreover, a consistent objectivist will be open-minded. Those who say that there are correct and incorrect answers in a given discipline must admit that possibly their answers are mistaken; for if the answers lie in the evidence external to the one making the judgment, then those individuals must admit that they could have gotten it wrong. Not all objectivists are open-minded; but that some objectivists are dogmatic is a problem with particular people, not with the position of objectivism. Similarly, objectivism might support tolerance. A meaningful principle of tolerance will say that agents *ought not* to impose their views on others. If that is true, it is a moral truth. Only objectivism allows for ultimate *moral* truths, so only objectivism can support a meaningful principle of tolerance.

This fifth argument for subjectivism is so popular that a further word about it is in order. One way to explain the argument's appeal is this. The promotion of open-mindedness and tolerance, many will agree, are admirable goals. Accepting subjectivism *seems* to promote these goals because subjectivism is, as it were, the great equalizer. If subjectivism is true, all moral beliefs and systems are equal. And if all beliefs and systems are recognized to be equal, it seems natural to think that open-mindedness and tolerance will follow. The problem, however, is that subjectivism purchases equality for conflicting moral beliefs at too high a price. According to subjectivism, all moral beliefs and systems are equal because none is true, in the sense of being binding on someone whether she accepts it or not. Once this is recognized, there is no good reason for subjectivists to be open-minded—to be willing to listen to the views and criticisms of others—because nothing else another says can convince subjectivists that their moral beliefs are false. Respect for conflicting views will come, it seems, only if one seriously entertains the possibility that those views, rather than one's own, may be correct. And this attitude, while compatible with objectivism, is not one that subjectivists can recommend.

It is sometimes claimed that one cannot prove or disprove moral judgments in the way that one can prove or disprove scientific judgments. This point is a sixth reason given to support subjectivism. Stated as a full argument, it reads:

6a. If judgments in an area cannot be proved or disproved, that area is subjective.
6b. Moral judgments cannot be proved or disproved.
6c. Therefore, morality is subjective.

Of the familiar arguments for subjectivism, this one is probably the most convincing. It raises several important questions. Are moral judgments different from scientific ones? If so, how? And are they different in such a way that leads to the justifiable conclusion that objectivism holds in the sciences but not in ethics? The answers to these questions are not obvious. Nevertheless, the objectivist can respond to this sixth argument in two ways.

The first point challenges the truth of premise 6a. On reflection, it seems clear that not all true statements can be proved and not all false statements can be disproved. Consider a statement about the distant past: It rained on the plain in Spain exactly 5,000 years ago. This statement is either true or false, and so objective in our sense. Yet no one can prove this statement if it is true, nor disprove it if it is false. Premise 6a is false because provability or disprovability is not necessary for objectivity.

The second point challenges the assertion in premise 6b. One might grant that moral judgments cannot be proved or disproved in the same way that scientific judgments are, but to assume that there is only one way to assess judgments is false. When we have different fields of inquiry, it seems reasonable to expect different methods of assessment. Consider history. Judgments in this field cannot be proved or disproved in the same way that scientific judgments are proved or disproved. For the key to assessing scientific judgments, we often hear, is repeatability; but obviously particular historical events are not repeatable. Or consider the law. Judges "prove" their opinions in that they provide reasoned discourse in support of them. But their method of citing explicit statutes, constitutional principles, and precedent is hardly what we call scientific. This point still leaves unanswered what proof in ethics is like, and it is appropriate to press on this issue. But to insist that all methods of proof be the same seems unwarranted.

Arguments for Objectivism

Suppose that you believe everything that you have read in this book so far. Does that give you any reason to believe that moral judgments are objective? It does not. All that we have done so far is to criticize the usual reasons given to support subjectivism. At this point, you may be agnostic; you may have no good reasons to support subjectivism, but also no good reasons to support objectivism. Several positive arguments in support of objectivism will now be presented. These arguments are designed to support the modest conclusion that most people believe or are committed to believing that moral judgments are objective.

The first argument, A1, may be stated as follows:

A1. 1. **Moral disputes do occur, situations in which each disputant tries to convince the other to adopt his or her position on the moral question at issue.**

2. When moral disputes occur, we—participants and spectators—do not ordinarily regard these activities as silly or irrational. On the contrary, we think that they are quite serious.

3. But if we believed that subjectivism were true, then we would regard moral disputes as silly or irrational.

4. Therefore, subjectivism conflicts with one of our basic beliefs about the moral life.

Argument A1 will be convincing only if each of the premises is plausible. Premises 1 and 2 are surely correct and need no defense. But why should one accept premise 3? It seems that subjectivists must say that moral disputes not rooted in factual disagreement are silly or irrational. It makes no sense for two people to argue about a matter to which there can, in principle, be no correct answer. Notice how we would regard a dispute about whether a certain flavor of ice cream is really good. This matter is clearly subjective, and debating it is pointless. And it should be clear that objectivists *can* explain why moral disputes are neither silly nor irrational: the disputants are seeking the correct answers to important questions.

Subjectivists may still insist that premise 3 is false. To defend this claim, subjectivists might argue that moral disputes, unlike debates about the goodness of a certain flavor of ice cream, have important consequences for the losers. People act on their moral beliefs, and their actions affect others. Suppose, for example, that your society is considering whether to institute capital punishment and you are opposed to such a practice. If you lose this debate, if your society does adopt capital punishment, this outcome can have adverse effects on your interests, especially if you are convicted of a capital offense! In such a case, when others act on a moral belief that you do not hold, you can be harmed. The same can be true if you take a person's privacy to be an important right while others put no value on this. Thus, subjectivists argue, moral disputes make sense, not because there are right answers to such questions but rather because people must look out for their own interests.

This response shows that subjectivists can explain why some moral disputes are appropriately regarded as neither silly nor irrational; but by no means does this explanation fit all of the cases. Those who oppose a moral belief even though they do not believe that either they or their loved ones will be harmed if others act on that belief are behaving irrationally, according to this view. So, if someone opposes voluntary euthanasia, not because that person believes that bad consequences will ensue from its adoption (and hence potential harm to herself) but rather because of the nature of the act, that person is behaving in a silly or irrational manner. The same must be said of those who oppose abortion with the consent of the pregnant woman, and of those who regard prostitution as wrong, again, when the basis of these judgments is not that bad consequences for others will follow from such acts. In neither of these cases do people regard their own interests as being threatened. Yet to conclude that their behavior is silly or irrational is surely too extreme. Even if we regard those who oppose voluntary euthanasia, abortion on request, and prostitution as misguided, we surely do not think that the very act of arguing against these practices is irrational. Hence, premise 3, properly qualified, is true.

Some might object that argument A1 merely shows that we do not *believe* that subjectivism is true; and since this belief might be false, we have no strict proof of objectivism. This, of course, is correct. But that does not mean that argument A1 is unimportant. A1 is an argument designed to shift the burden of proof. It is fashioned to show how radically at odds with our ordinary beliefs about the moral life subjectivism is. Since any adequate metaethical theory must account for fundamental beliefs about the moral life and the common usage of moral terms, this casts doubt on subjectivism. At the very least the onus is on the subjectivist to show why the ordinary view of moral disputes is mistaken.

A second argument to support objectivism appeals to the way that people regard the behavior of agents facing difficult moral problems:

A2. 1. **Moral predicaments do occur, situations in which the agents believe that they have reasons for doing each of two actions both of which they cannot do, and the agents do not know which is more important.**

2. **When agents are in moral predicaments, they often seek moral advice.**

3. **That agents seek advice in such situations seems appropriate, certainly not silly or irrational.**

4. **But if we believed that subjectivism were true, we would regard seeking moral advice as silly or irrational.**

5. **Therefore, subjectivism conflicts with one of our basic beliefs about the moral life.**

Again, this argument will render the conclusion plausible only if the premises can be defended. The first three premises are uncontroversial; they merely involve observations about what goes on when people partake in the moral life. But premise 4, the crucial one, requires explanation. If an agent has examined all of the relevant facts, then subjectivism implies that there is nothing to seek advice about. Recall that the subjectivist says that answers to moral questions are neither correct nor incorrect. As a result, the subjectivist must regard seeking advice about ethical issues as being on a par with asking someone else what flavor of ice cream really tastes good. In either case, the question is pointless; for, by hypothesis, nothing that the other person says can help one make a more rational decision.

Subjectivists may wish to reject premise 4. They may argue that it is not silly, inappropriate, or irrational to consult with others about moral matters because acting on such beliefs has serious consequences. People must come to an agreement with each other about moral beliefs to avoid disastrous consequences. Note, for example, how chaotic and miserable life would be if people did not generally agree that killing and stealing are wrong. Thus, even though moral issues cannot be resolved rationally, it makes sense to consult about such matters; doing so promotes social stability.

Again, however, this response applies to a limited range of cases. In a number of other situations, people appropriately seek moral advice even though the subjectivist's explanation is inapplicable. Consider, for example, a person contemplating suicide. The consequences for society need not be disastrous if there is no general agreement concerning this issue. Yet we think that people considering suicide are behaving quite appropriately if they seek advice before acting. And such people's behavior is no less appropriate if they have no relatives who might suffer or be harmed by a successful suicide. It seems, then, that subjectivists must say that seeking advice in situations like this is inappropriate. Such a contention, however, is not plausible. So, in spite of subjectivists' objection, premise 4 of argument A2 holds for a large number of cases, which is all that objectivists need.

A third argument for objectivism appeals to the way that agents often behave after they have faced difficult moral situations, and it may be sketched as follows:

A3. 1. **People sometimes experience moral doubt after they have acted.**

2. **That people experience moral doubt seems appropriate, and certainly not irrational.**

3. **But if we believed that subjectivism were true, we would normally regard experiencing moral doubt as inappropriate or irrational.**

4. **Therefore, subjectivism conflicts with one of our basic beliefs about the moral life.**

The first two premises of this argument are self-explanatory and surely plausible; they merely involve observations about the behavior of people engaged in normative ethics. Premise 3, however, requires explanation. Under normal circumstances, subjectivists must regard experiencing moral doubt as irrational or inappropriate. The reason for this is that individuals cannot doubt whether what they have done was really right or wrong when, by hypothesis, no actions are really right or wrong. Doubt is an appropriate attitude only when individuals can be mistaken, and subjectivists are committed to saying that there is no such thing as a purely moral mistake.

Subjectivists might retort that the reason that doubt about moral matters is appropriate is that the individual is worried about the practical consequences of being assessed negatively by members of society. This retaliation may take the form of moral censure or something more severe, such as incarceration. That doubt is regarded as appropriate, then, can be explained by subjectivists. There is a difficulty, though. However plausible this response may seem, it cannot begin to explain adequately all cases. Having had an abortion, a woman may question whether she has done the right thing even though she believes that no one else will find out about this act. The source of her worry is not that she will be blamed by her society, yet we do not regard her doubt as irrational. This and similar examples show that premise 3 of argument A3 is true of a number of cases; thus, the subjectivist's response is inadequate.

Let us consider one other argument for objectivism, one designed to show that many cannot accept the consequences of subjectivism:

A4. 1. **If we believed that subjectivism were true, then the only way that we could legitimately criticize someone else's moral views would be to show that they are internally inconsistent.**

   2. **So if we believed that subjectivism were true, then we could not criticize the moral views of someone like Hitler, assuming that his views are consistent.**

   3. **But we do want to say that there is something wrong with Hitler's moral views, even if they are consistent.**

   4. **Therefore, most of us cannot accept the consequences of subjectivism.**

A brief explanation of premise 1 is in order. Subjectivists can say negative things about the moral views of others even if they believe that those views are consistent. But subjectivists cannot regard themselves as trying to show that these other views are mistaken. After all, according to subjectivism, morality is not the sort of thing about which one can be ultimately mistaken. Instead, when subjectivists say negative things about others' moral views, they must regard themselves as being engaged in a war of propaganda, as it were. In criticizing others' views on ethical matters, people are not trying to show that those views are wrong; rather, they are simply trying to get others to adopt their favorite position. But is that what one is really doing when one criticizes the moral views of someone like Hitler? Consistent, hard-nosed subjectivists may be willing to say this. But such a response seems inadequate; most of us think that there is something mistaken—something morally wrong—with Hitler's views.

These four arguments have a modest aim. They are merely designed to show how fundamentally subjectivism conflicts with widely held beliefs about the moral life. It is possible, of course, that these widely held beliefs are mistaken. But the burden of proof is on subjectivists. For when a position conflicts with common sense, proponents of that position must show us why we should abandon common sense. So, we have good reasons to hold, at least tentatively, that morality is objective.

GENERAL PRINCIPLES

If morality is objective—if there are right and wrong answers to moral questions—then it is important to ask what the criteria are for determining these matters. Here we shall discuss three basic moral principles and then outline two major ethical theories.

For any area of professional ethics, it is important to begin by distinguishing between general obligations and role-related obligations. *General obligations* are moral requirements that agents have simply because they are moral agents. That moral agents are required not to kill, not to steal, and not to rape are examples of general obligations; each agent is bound by these requirements. By contrast, *role-related obligations* are moral requirements that agents have by virtue of their role, occupation, or position in society. That lifeguards are required to save swimmers in distress, that teachers are required to educate their students, and that physicians are required to provide reliable medical care for their patients are examples of role-related obligations. It might be, of course, that anyone who is in a position to do so ought to save a drowning person. Certainly if you could save someone's life merely by tossing a life preserver, you ought to do so. But lifeguards have obligations to help swimmers in distress even when most others do not because of their abilities and contractual commitments.

As we shall see, many of the issues in medical ethics involve conflicts between commonly acknowledged general obligations and role-related obligations. Occasionally in the context of professional ethics, someone will argue that in cases of conflict, role-related obligations should always take precedence over general obligations. As we shall see, this claim is dubious. A far more plausible contention is that in cases of conflict, sometimes general obligations override role-related obligations and sometimes role-related obligations override general obligations. Examples will be given throughout this book to demonstrate this point. We shall also see that role-related obligations can conflict because people typically occupy more than one role. For example, a physician may also be a parent, a member of the school board, and president of the county medical society. Each of these roles carries with it obligations, and such obligations may conflict. We shall also see that obligations attached to the same role may conflict. A physician's obligation to one patient may conflict with an obligation to a second patient. How best to resolve such conflicts is a major part of medical ethics.

Let us now briefly discuss three moral principles acknowledged by many to be general obligations and the basis for many role-related obligations.[2] The *principle of nonmaleficence* says that moral agents ought not to inflict evil or harm on others. The requirements not to kill, not to steal, and not to rape are based on this more general principle. Those who say that a health care practitioner's first maxim should be "Above all, do no harm" are affirming the centrality of this principle. Breaching the confidence of a patient is wrong, in part, because such activity may harm the patient.

The *principle of autonomy* says that moral agents ought not to interfere with the actions and choices of other autonomous individuals. Physically detaining someone against that person's will violates the principle of autonomy. Deceiving another often violates this principle since deception is one way of manipulating another's choices. Breaching a patient's confidence may be wrong not only because it harms the patient but also because it violates that individual's autonomy, assuming that the patient has the right to determine who has access to personal information.

The *principle of beneficence* says that moral agents ought to promote the welfare of others. This principle is complicated in at least two ways, however. First, promoting the welfare of others may take different forms. It may involve preventing harm, such as when someone pulls a drowning child from the pool. It may involve removing harm, such as when someone gives another medication to cure an illness. Or it may involve positively contributing to another's good, such as when someone provides another with a gift. The second complication concerns the "other" for whom assistance is provided. That other may be a particular individual for whom one has a special responsibility, such as a child or a client. That other may be an institution to which one is closely related, such as a hospital or a university. Or that other may be any third party to whom one has no special obligations.

Not only can conflicts occur between general obligations and role-related obligations, but they can also emerge between/among the three principles just explained. For example, a health care practitioner may be tempted to violate a patient's autonomy to promote that patient's welfare. Again, a major concern in this book is how best to resolve these conflicts.

As was indicated earlier, normative ethics has different levels of specificity. You are engaged in normative ethics if you are deliberating about what you ought to do in a specific situation. You are also engaged in normative ethics if you articulate and defend basic moral rules and principles, such as those discussed previously. Normative ethics can be pursued at an even higher level of abstraction, however. Suppose you think that lying to a patient about a medical condition is wrong and that breaching the confidence of a patient is wrong. It is reasonable to ask what is it that makes both of these types of actions wrong. And if you think that people should not harm others, should respect the autonomy of others, and should sometimes assist others in need, it is natural to ask what is it that makes all of these actions right. When we attempt to say what characteristics are shared by all and only right actions, or when we try to isolate the features shared by all and only wrong actions, we are practicing normative ethics at the highest level of generality.

ETHICAL THEORIES

Conflicting answers to these broad questions have been advanced, and they can be divided into two general theories about what makes an action right/wrong: consequentialism and deontologism. Each of these theories will be explained next, and their relevance to the central issues of medical ethics will be addressed throughout this book.

Consequentialism

Consequentialist moral theories hold that the rightness or wrongness of actions is determined solely by the results those actions produce. The inherent nature of an action is not morally relevant. The only factor that counts in the moral assessment of an action is the value of that action's consequences. In its precise formulation, consequentialism says that an act is right if and only if it produces consequences at least as good as the consequences of any alternative act open to the agent. Put more simply, consequentialists say that agents facing a moral situation should do the following: determine the alternative acts that can be performed in that situation, estimate the consequences, both good and bad, that are likely to result from the performance of each act, and then perform that act that is likely to have the best consequences on balance. Consequentialists affirm the familiar maxim that the end justifies the means.

Though putting it this way is oversimplified, we could say that consequentialists instruct moral agents to maximize the good. But whose good should be maximized? On this point, consequentialists disagree among themselves, leading to different versions of that general theory.

One version of consequentialism, *ethical egoism*, says that each agent should maximize his own interests only. Egoism is not significant in biomedical ethics, so it will not be discussed here.

At the other end of the consequentialist spectrum is *utilitarianism*. Utilitarianism requires agents to perform those actions that bring about the greatest balance of good over evil in the universe as a whole; more simply, utilitarianism instructs agents to maximize the good of all affected parties. For our purposes here, we need to distinguish further two versions of utilitarianism.

According to *act utilitarianism*, agents should appeal directly to the principle of utility each time they make a moral decision. More precisely, act utilitarianism says that an act is right if and only if that act produces consequences at least as good for all affected parties as the consequences of any alternative act open to the agent. Suppose that a physician has diagnosed Juan as having a terminal illness and wonders whether to be truthful with him about this condition. Act utilitarianism says that the physician should note the alternative acts available, determine the likely consequences of each alternative for everyone affected, and perform that act that in this situation results in the best balance of good over evil considering everyone affected. If tomorrow this same physician wonders whether to be truthful with Maria about her terminal illness, the calculations must be done anew; for what maximizes the good in one situation may not do so in another. To use a concept introduced earlier, act utilitarianism allows for context dependence.

Act utilitarianism is often difficult to apply in particular situations because agents may lack knowledge of the likely consequences of their acts or may have no time to calculate. This leads us to consider an alternative form of utilitarianism. According to *rule utilitarianism*, agents should appeal to a set of moral rules each time they make a moral decision. These moral rules should be established on the basis of the principle of utility. Whether a rule is part of the set to which an agent should appeal depends on whether everyone's adopting it will result in better consequences than everyone's adopting some different rule. More precisely, rule utilitarianism says that an act is right if and only if that act is in accord with a set of moral rules, the general acceptance of which will have consequences at least as good for all affected parties as the consequences of everyone's adopting some other set of rules. Agents employing this theory appeal to the principle of utility only indirectly. Once the ideal rules are in place, further appeal to the principle of utility is unnecessary, except possibly when two rules conflict. If rule utilitarianism instructs the physician in the previous example to be truthful with Juan about his terminal illness, it will also instruct that physician to be honest with Maria.

As we shall see, when we examine particular moral issues, an appeal to utilitarian considerations is natural. Indeed, there are obvious connections between the principle of beneficence, so central in medicine, and utilitarianism. We shall also see that rule utilitarian considerations are often cited to justify what laws should be enacted.

Egoism, which advocates that each agent maximize his own good, and utilitarianism, which counsels agents to maximize the good of the whole, are not the only consequentialist theories. For some theories advocate maximizing the good for some selected group of individuals. Nationalist or racist theories may be understood in this way, though they are of little interest in medical ethics. What is of interest here, though, is a theory that we shall call *patient (client) consequentialism*. According to this view, health care practitioners, when acting in their professional roles, always ought to do that which has the best overall results for their patients (clients). James Gregory, a teaching physician at the medical school in Edinburgh, Scotland, expressed such a view in 1800:

> Whatever was best for the physician's patients, it was his indispensable duty to do for them. Whatever was bad, or unnecessarily dangerous for them, it was his duty not to do; and both these duties were with him supreme and indefeasible.[3]

Codes of ethics in the various medical fields also sometimes express such an outlook. Notice that patient consequentialism urges that one's role-related obligations as a health care practitioner always take precedence over any obligations with which they might conflict. Because of the prevalence of this view, we shall discuss its implications for the various issues presented in this book. We should note, however, that three types of cases raise potential problems for patient consequentialism: (1) when doing what is in the patient's best interests adversely affects innocent third parties, (2) when the patient is unwilling to do what the health care practitioner judges is in that patient's best interests, and (3) when doing what is in one patient's best interests adversely affects the interests of another patient.

Deontologism

Not everyone agrees with the moral outlook of the consequentialist. Nonconsequentialist views are usually called *deontological moral theories*. Put simply, deontologists hold that the moral status of an action is *not* determined *solely* by the value of the consequences that act produces. You might wonder what else could be relevant in assessing an action. Deontologists sometimes say that the kind of action that an agent performs is also morally relevant. The inherent nature of an action, as well as the consequences it produces, can make a moral difference. Consequentialists are concerned only with what happens or what state of affairs is produced. As long as the greatest good is brought about, it does not matter who the agents were or what sort of acts they performed. By contrast, deontologists are concerned not only with what happens but also with what people do; the nature of an agent's act is morally important. Deontologists maintain that there are moral limits on what one may do in the pursuit of good consequences. Certain things may not be done merely because they maximize the good; examples may include killing an innocent person, torturing a human being, or knowingly punishing an innocent individual. Deontologists, then, deny that the end justifies the means.

To clarify the differences between consequentialist and deontological reasoning, consider the following (nonmedical) case.

Suppose that a Nazi war criminal responsible for the torture and deaths of many innocent people escaped in 1945. He was a high-ranking officer in the Nazi army, so it was deemed important to capture and punish him. The pursuit of him, however, was unsuccessful. For the past thirty years he has been living incognito in a South American village. He has become a useful and prosperous member of the community; indeed, he has been a model citizen. In 1980, because of the work of an investigative reporter, the identity and whereabouts of this war criminal, now seventy years old, are made known. Should this man be punished? If so, how?

Some people say that the Nazi should not be punished. It will serve no good purpose, they say. When pressed, they are apt to claim that the main purposes of punishment are to minimize crime by incarcerating criminals, rehabilitate the criminal, and deter others from committing similar crimes. In short, these people reason as consequentialists in general, and utilitarians in particular. And it is their contention that no good consequences will result from punishing the Nazi since he is apparently already rehabilitated and war crimes are difficult to deter. By contrast, others will claim that the Nazi should be punished. He violated the rights of others by forcibly detaining them, torturing them, and in some cases killing them. He has thereby forfeited some of his own rights, and justice demands that he be punished, regardless of whether doing so produces good consequences. Persons taking this position are arguing from a deontological perspective.

Rights When issues in ethics and political philosophy are debated, participants frequently appeal to the notion of rights. Talk about rights is pervasive in medical ethics too. Indeed, one of the frustrating things is that it seems that all sides on all issues invoke rights to support their case. Consider, as one example, the issue of abortion. Supporters of the so-called "pro-choice" position appeal to a woman's right to make her own medical decisions to defend their position. And advocates of the so-called "pro-life" position appeal to the fetus's right to life to support their view. Many controversial issues arise about rights, and the philosophical and legal literature on these topics is extensive. Here we shall merely make some brief remarks about the concept of a *right*. As with general moral theories, our understanding of rights will emerge gradually within the context of specific issues.

A person's rights affect the moral status of others' actions. Rights are valuable moral commodities that put legitimate restraints on how others may act toward the person who possesses the rights. If one person has a right, others have obligations or duties with respect to that person. A defining characteristic of rights is that they imply duties or obligations on others (sometimes referred to as correlative obligations).

Two bases for distinctions among rights are on the *content* of the correlative obligation and *on whom* the correlative obligation falls. If the correlative obligation is to provide goods or services to the possessor, then the right is said to be *positive*. If a child has a right to be educated, for instance, such a right is positive. If the correlative obligation is to refrain from doing something, then the right is said to be *negative*. For example, if people have a right not to be tortured, it is negative; it puts obligations on others not to do certain things. The correlative obligations associated with some rights fall on all moral agents; these rights are universal (or *in rem*). An example is a person's right to life; such a right puts obligations on all other moral agents. The correlative obligation associated with other rights are restricted (or *in personam*); these obligations fall only on selected individuals. If Maria promised Tony that she would help him move this afternoon, Tony has a right to assistance that places obligations only on Maria. Some say that a child has a right to be nurtured and that this right places obligations only on the child's parents.

Some say that rights provide protection for individuals against utility-maximizing claims; so understood, rights put restrictions on what society may do to promote the overall good. When rights are characterized in this way, their natural place seems to be within a deontological theory. This *characterization* is because consequentialists, it seems, must endorse the rightness of any action that will produce the best balance of good over evil in the circumstances. And the act that produces the best overall consequences in some circumstances may violate the rights of someone. Though this view is the common way of looking at things, we should note that some believe that consequentialist moral theories can accommodate rights; indeed, some think that consequentialist theories can make better sense of rights than can deontological theories.[4] So, though appeals to rights are common, it is fair to say that no consensus prevails on what the moral foundation for those rights is.

MORAL PROBLEMS

As we discuss particular issues, such as confidentiality, truth telling, and treatment without consent, we shall see that conflicts between consequentialist and deontological considerations are frequent. These and the other issues we discuss are among the moral problems that arise in medical contexts.

A *moral problem* is a situation in which there are moral considerations to support one action, say act A; moral considerations to support another action, act B; and act A and act B cannot both be done. Situations like this are morally problematic if agents facing them do not know, at least initially, which of the competing considerations are more important. Agents encountering such situations deliberate in an attempt to resolve the moral problems.

Some believe that many of the moral problems encountered in medical contexts are irresolvable. The allusion here is not to the subjectivist, who says that there are no correct answers to moral questions; rather, the reference is to those who say that there are genuine moral dilemmas. A *genuine moral dilemma* is a situation in which an agent really ought to do each of two acts, but doing both acts is impossible. No matter what choice the agent makes, that person will have done something wrong or failed to do something that he ought to have done. An agent facing a moral dilemma is, in one sense, morally doomed. Moral dilemmas are *irresolvable* moral problems. No further moral deliberation will help agents who are in dilemmas.

Many agonizing moral problems exist. Whether some of these are irresolvable in principle is a matter of debate.[5]

The principal goals in this text are to identify some of the main moral problems that arise in medicine and to explain the moral considerations that support conflicting alternatives. Sometimes solutions to the problems will be endorsed, and not all readers will agree with them. That discord, however, is healthy; for only by engaging in ongoing debate can we hope to resolve some of these difficult issues.

SUMMARY

As noted at the outset, the particular issues discussed in this book fall in the realm of normative ethics. The principal focus of this chapter, however, has been on the dispute between subjectivists and objectivists, a dispute concerning a fundamental issue in metaethics. The arguments supporting subjectivism are seriously flawed because they assume that features such as the existence of widespread disagreement, the absence of uncertainty about particular cases, and the lack of provability demonstrate that there are no correct answers to moral questions. But because each of these characteristics is also associated with areas widely believed to be objective, the principal assumptions of these arguments appear to be false. And while the arguments favoring objectivism are not conclusive, they shift the burden of proof; they show that objectivism fits better with common beliefs about the moral life.

Two general normative theories—consequentialism and deontologism—were introduced. Consequentialists hold that an act is right just in case it produces consequences at least as good as the consequences of any alternative acts. But good for whom? Utilitarianism counsels agents to bring about the best possible consequences for all affected parties. Patient consequentialism directs health professionals to focus only on the interests of those to whom they are providing care. Deontologists, on the other hand, deny that results alone are the basis for judging the rightness of acts; they say that additional factors, such as individual rights, must be taken into account in the moral assessment of acts.

As we examine particular moral problems that arise in the delivery of health care, we shall see the relevance of these various theoretical considerations.

Suggestions for Further Reading

Beauchamp, Tom L., and James F. Childress. *Principles of Biomedical Ethics*, 4th ed. (New York: Oxford University Press, 1994), Chapters 1 and 2.

Beauchamp, Tom L., and LeRoy Walters (eds.). *Contemporary Issues in Bioethics*, 4th ed. (Belmont, CA: Wadsworth, 1994), Chapter 1.

Rachels, James. *The Elements of Moral Philosophy* (New York: McGraw-Hill, 1986), Chapters 1, 2, 3, and 8.

Notes

1. For a detailed discussion of this argument, see Terrance McConnell, "Objectivity and Moral Expertise," *Canadian Journal of Philosophy*, Vol. 14 (1984), pp. 193–216.

2. For a detailed discussion of these principles and their role in medical ethics, see Tom L. Beauchamp and James F. Childress, *Principles of Biomedical Ethics*, 4th ed. (New York: Oxford University Press, 1994), Chapters 3, 4, and 5.

Throughout this book I emphasize the role of these principles in the specific issues discussed. Some have called such a view "principlism" and have been critical of it. For a discussion of those criticisms and responses to them, see Beauchamp and Childress, pp. 104–108. For a brief discussion of alternatives to principlism in clinical contexts, see George A. Kanoti and Stuart Younger, "Clinical Ethics Consultation," in Warren Reich (ed.), *Encyclopedia of Bioethics*, rev. ed. (Upper Saddle River, NJ: Prentice Hall, 1995), Vol. 1, pp. 404–409. See also Søren Holm, "Not Just Autonomy—The Principles of American Biomedical Ethics," *Journal of Medical Ethics*, Vol. 21 (1995), pp. 332–338.

3. Quoted in Mary Ann Carroll and Richard A. Humphrey, *Moral Problems in Nursing: Case Studies* (Washington, D.C.: University Press of America, 1979), p. 15.

4. See L. W. Sumner, *The Moral Foundations of Rights* (New York: Oxford University Press, 1987).

5. For an excellent collection of essays on this issue representing diverse points of view, see Christopher W. Gowans (ed.), *Moral Dilemmas* (New York: Oxford University Press, 1987).

CHAPTER 2

Moral Problems in the Health Care Practitioner– Patient Relationship

SEVERAL MORAL ISSUES ARISE in the context of the one-to-one relationship between health care practitioners and patients. One general issue concerns the way in which the relationship between health care professionals and patients should be conceived. Different models of that relationship will be discussed here, and moral differences among them will be highlighted. After that, two particular moral problems will be addressed. The first concerns the confidentiality of communications between health care practitioners and patients. Are there any conditions under which health care workers may justifiably breach this confidence? If so, what are they? The second concerns being honest with patients about their own medical conditions. Is it ever permissible for health care professionals to withhold the truth from patients about their own medical conditions? If so, when?

MODELS OF THE HEALTH CARE PRACTITIONER–PATIENT RELATIONSHIP

The very way that health care professionals envision their relationship with patients can have significant ethical implications. And though this topic may seem abstract, in fact it has important practical import. How health care workers conceive their roles in relation to patients will affect all of the moral decisions they make in that context. Robert M.

Veatch has discussed three dominant models of the health care practitioner–patient relationship.[1] Each of these models articulates an *ideal* of how the relationship should be regarded. No defender of any of the models would claim that the relationship always exists as it ought to be. In the real world, things are far more muddled.

Engineering Model

According to this model, health care professionals should regard themselves as applied scientists. So conceived, they must deal only with facts and divorce themselves from all questions of value. The role of physicians, for example, is to present the facts to patients, and then let them make their own decisions. Physicians are to make no value judgments about their patients' decisions. Or, more accurately, physicians must not let their value judgments affect their actions in medical contexts. In this view, then, a Roman Catholic physician, who in his private life believes that abortion is murder, should have no qualms about performing an abortion for a patient who requests it. This is his role as an applied scientist. A desirable feature of the engineering model is that it views patients as autonomous beings capable of making their own decisions; it respects the principle of autonomy. But there are three undesirable features of this model, and together they suggest that this is not an appropriate way to conceive the patient–health care practitioner relationship.

First, it is impossible for health care workers not to make and act on moral judgments—not because of emotional considerations. Rather, all people are put in situations where they must make and act on value judgments, and this is especially true in the field of medicine. Consider the following scenario. A man comes to his physician with medical problems. Various tests are performed, and among other things the man learns that he is HIV-positive. The man is engaged to be married. The physician tells the man that it is important that he inform his fiancée about his condition and that he either abstain from sexual intercourse or engage in only so-called safe sex. The man says that he will not change his sexual practices and will not inform his fiancée. The physician wonders whether she should breach confidence and warn the woman. This physician is faced with a moral problem, one that is increasingly familiar today. Whatever decision she makes, it is a moral decision. Avoiding morality is not an option here, which is true in many situations.

Second, expecting health care professionals to participate in acts that privately they believe are immoral is unfair and undesirable. It is unfair because it says to them that their own moral views do not count and that they should have no qualms about violating them. It is undesirable because we do not want to encourage people to perform acts that they believe are wrong or to take a cavalier attitude toward morality. In the example of the Roman Catholic physician, surely we do not want to encourage him to perform acts that he believes are murder. We risk creating a moral schizophrenic.

Third, patients may ask physicians to provide them with drugs or treatments that will harm those patients, and it is far from obvious that health care practitioners should comply with such requests. Patients hooked on addictive prescription drugs may demand more and more. The engineering model suggests that physicians should comply with their wishes. This case brings to the fore the underlying problem. The engineering model emphasizes patient autonomy but gives no weight to beneficence.

The engineering model presents itself as value-neutral. But, as these criticisms show, it is not evaluatively neutral. The very essence of this model—to present all of the facts and let patients decide—is itself a moral position. The engineering model, then, does not present an attractive ideal in conceptualizing the patient–health care worker relationship.

Paternalistic Model

Veatch refers to this as the "priestly" model. According to this model, patients come to health care practitioners for treatment, counsel, and comfort. The ideal portrayed here is that decision making is placed entirely in the hands of health care professionals, and patients are expected to follow their orders. One assumes that health care workers *know* what is best for patients and *will* do what is best for them. The slogan associated with this model is "Benefit and do no harm to the patient." While attacking this principle might initially seem absurd, its implications are troubling.

One criticism of this model, Veatch suggests, is that it involves an inappropriate generalization of expertise. What he means by this is that the model inadvertently depicts health care providers as having expertise in areas where they do not. Their expertise is in technical matters. Yet not all decisions in medical contexts are merely technical; as noted earlier, sometimes the decisions are moral. This model says that health care practitioners are to make all decisions because they know what is best and will do what is best. But while they may know what is *medically* best for patients, they may not know what is overall best. Veatch says that this transference of expertise is sometimes signaled by the "speaking-as-a . . ." syndrome.[2] Thus, a physician may preface advice by saying, "Speaking as your physician, I recommend . . . ." This statement gives what is said an aura of authority. But if what follows involves moral advice, the physician may not be an authority. Veatch's example here concerns a pregnant woman who has taken Thalidomide. If her physician informs her that the odds are against a normal baby and that this is a risk she should not take, the advice has gone beyond merely technical matters. The more general point is that many decisions in medical contexts are like this.

A second criticism of this model is that it gives health care workers too much power. Put more baldly, this model is too paternalistic. There are simply some decisions that competent patients must make for themselves. Decisions concerning amputation of limbs and sterilization, for example, have an enormous impact on a person's life; how anyone other than the affected person could make decisions about such matters is difficult to fathom.

The paternalistic model emphasizes beneficence at the expense of autonomy. It counsels health care professionals to do what is best for their patients without regard to the wishes of those patients.

Contractual Model

This model of the relationship between patients and health care providers attempts to capture desirable features of the previous two models. The principal features of this model may be summarized as follows. First, the relationship between patients and health care providers is best conceived as an implied, tacit contract between the two. The relationship involves a true sharing, and each party has a role to play in the decision-making process.

Second, each party has obligations, and each party can be expected to derive benefits. Health care workers are obligated to provide patients with information about their options and to recommend what they judge will be best. Patients are expected to provide physicians and nurses with all of the information about their condition they are aware of and to follow the plan of treatment mutually agreed on. Each party is required to be honest with the other. The expected benefits for patients are comfort and a return to good health, if possible; health care professionals will accrue monetary rewards and professional satisfaction. Obligations of patients are seldom emphasized. But the contractual model conceives the relationship as mutual and noncompliant patients are not upholding their end.

Third, patients are free to make all significant decisions. Their fully informed consent must be obtained before treatment is initiated.

Fourth, day-to-day technical decisions may be made by health care practitioners. As long as the patient agrees with the general goal and has not forbidden some particular means, health care workers may make technical decisions necessary to implement that goal. Admittedly, however, the line between major decisions and technical ones may be blurry.

Finally, if agreement cannot be reached, each party is free to end the relationship in a timely manner. Of course, if patients are dissatisfied with the services rendered, they may go elsewhere. But health care providers have this same freedom. If, for example, a physician has strong objections to a request made by a patient, it would be unfair to demand that the physician honor that request. Ending a relationship because of a moral disagreement can be quite problematic; clearly it is better if the issue can be resolved.[3] These difficulties can be minimized if each party is open and honest at all times. Thus, a patient who has religious objections to blood transfusions should make this known to the physician at the outset. And if a physician is never willing to discontinue life support, patients should be so informed.

The contractual model attempts to satisfy both autonomy and beneficence. Because it ultimately allows patients to make final decisions, it gives priority to autonomy. But it acknowledges that the role of health care practitioners is to help patients, and it does not demand of these professionals that they do anything that patients want. What we have is beneficence constrained by autonomy.

The values of patients and health care practitioners can and sometimes do conflict. Each of these three models resolves such conflicts differently. The engineering model resolves all such conflicts in favor of patients, requiring health care practitioners to ignore their own values. The paternalistic model resolves these conflicts in favor of health care workers, ignoring what patients may want. The contractual model attempts to respect the views of all involved; it requires that the parties agree and, if they cannot, that the relationship be ended.

The paternalistic model is appropriate in some obvious contexts. If the patient lacks the capacity to make decisions—because, for example, of being unconscious, severely retarded, or not of age—then the patient is not in a position to exercise autonomy, and someone else must make those medical decisions. Of course, someone other than or in addition to the physician may be the appropriate decision maker; but it would seem that paternalism of some sort must enter the picture here.

Today the pendulum has swung from paternalism and to the contractual model, and in some contexts that approach is proper. When patients are competent and well educated, most will agree that in the end they must make their own decisions. We should acknowledge, however, that there are many situations in which these matters are muddled. For example, patients may be competent but not well positioned to make their own decisions. Suppose that a physician in a clinic treats mostly patients who are poorly educated, homeless, and addicted to alcohol. It may be a stretch to suppose that the contractual model is the best way to conceive the relationship between this doctor and the patients. On the other hand, pure paternalism may not be the proper way to conceive the relationship, either. Also, some competent patients prefer to be treated paternalistically. For various reasons, some patients are passive and fearful of making their own decisions; they prefer the "old-time" view of patients. Cases like these show some of the real-life complexities and demonstrate why these models are simply ideals.

In concluding this section, we should clarify one point about the contractual model. While in general it does not allow for paternalism, it does not compel health care practitioners to accede to all of the wishes of their patients. Thus, if a patient wants a treatment that a physician thinks is harmful or unwise, a physician is under no obligation to provide that treatment. Obvious examples include refusing to prescribe certain drugs or sterilize a patient. A physician's refusal in these cases may be paternalistic; the physician may think that the treatment or procedure will harm the patient. But this response is what one might call "negative" paternalism in that the physician is *refraining* from doing something. And because the contractual model respects the values of health care workers, too, it allows them to refuse to initiate treatments that they believe are not warranted.

CONFIDENTIALITY

Communications between patients and health care practitioners are supposed to be private. The content of such conversations, as well as what is learned about the patients, is to be conveyed only to others involved in the care of those patients. Confidentiality is fundamental to this relationship.

Confidentiality may be compromised in many ways and for different reasons. A health care worker might breach confidence out of spite or malice; such behavior is obviously wrong. More commonly, confidentiality may be undermined because of carelessness. Leaving confidential records open and unattended and talking about cases in crowded elevators are examples of such carelessness. Consider this mundane case: Tom was waiting in a crowded room while his wife was undergoing outpatient surgery. During the hour that Tom spent in the waiting room, five physicians entered and talked to relatives about surgeries performed on their family members. These conversations occurred within earshot of most of the people in the room. Tom heard nothing juicy or interesting that afternoon; indeed, later he remembered nothing specific that he had overheard. But Tom remembered one thing very well. When his wife's physician had completed the surgery and sought out Tom, he took him in the hall, beyond the earshot of others, before he told him about the outcome. This surgeon demonstrated an appropriate sensitivity about confidentiality that the first five lacked. This quality is important even if the content of the conversations is quite ordinary.

It should go without saying that confidentiality should not be compromised because of malice or carelessness. But from the moral point of view, the most important question is this: Are health care practitioners ever *morally justified* in breaching the confidence of a patient? If so, when and for what reasons? This question can be put another way: Is the confidentiality obligation *absolute?* Or are there legitimate exceptions? These are the questions that we shall focus on here.

Confidentiality and Codes of Medical Ethics

Most codes of medical ethics acknowledge the importance of confidentiality. And some suggest that the confidentiality obligation is absolute. For example, the Declaration of Geneva, written in 1948, says, "I will hold in confidence *all* that my patient confides in me."[4] And the International Code of Medical Ethics, devised by the World Medical Association in 1949, reads as follows: "A doctor owes to his patient *absolute* secrecy on *all* which has been confided to him or which he knows because of the confidence entrusted to him."

Other codes are less clear about the status of the confidentiality obligation. The best-known code of medical ethics is the Hippocratic Oath, and concerning confidentiality it states, "What I may see or hear in the course of the treatment or even outside of the treatment in regard to the life of men, which on no account one must speak abroad, I will keep to myself holding such things shameful to be spoken about." It is difficult to know what is intended here. Read one way, "which on no account one must speak abroad" refers to everything that a physician sees or hears in the course of treatment; read another way, it refers to a subset thereof. It is difficult to know which interpretation is more plausible.

Other codes of ethics are clearer. In 1959 the British Medical Association issued a statement that claimed that the rule of professional secrecy may be broken only under two conditions: (1) when statutory sanction will be imposed if the physician fails to disclose the information or (2) when breaching confidence will be in the best interests of the patient.[5]

On June 26, 1990, the American Medical Association House of Delegates adopted a report of the Council on Ethical and Judicial Affairs. Concerning confidentiality, the report said:

> The patient has the right to confidentiality. The physician should not reveal confidential communications or information without the consent of the patient, unless provided for by law or by the need to protect the welfare of the individual or the public interest.

This statement mirrors an earlier position endorsed by the AMA in its Principles of Medical Ethics (adopted in 1957 and revised in 1971):

> A physician may not reveal the confidences entrusted to him in the course of medical attendance, or the deficiencies he may observe in the character of his patients, unless he is required to do so by law or unless it becomes necessary to protect the welfare of the individual or of the society.[6]

So the AMA says that confidentiality may be breached when any one of three conditions obtains: (1) when breaching confidence is in the best interests of the individual patient, (2) when required by law to breach confidence, or (3) when breaching confidence is in the public interest.

Examples of each of the exceptions endorsed by the AMA will be helpful. The most obvious example of breaching confidence to protect the patient's own interests is the case of a potential suicide. If a health care professional has a patient whom she believes is a high risk for suicide, so informing family members may minimize the chances that such an act will be carried out. More generally, today many psychiatric patients are not being treated in an inpatient setting. As a result, family members bear a larger burden of care for these patients. Arguably both patients and the family members would be better off if certain otherwise confidential information were conveyed by the health care givers to the relevant family members.[7] And perhaps likely noncompliant patients would be better off if their family members were informed of their treatment regimen and so could cajole these patients to prevent noncompliance.

Laws vary from country to country, and within the United States from state to state. But typical examples in which health care professionals may be required to reveal information about patients include reporting prima facie evidence of child abuse to appropriate social agencies, reporting gunshot wounds treated, and reporting patients treated for certain contagious diseases, such as syphilis, gonorrhea, and tuberculosis.

There are many examples of breaching confidence to protect the public interest. One is the famous case of Richard Speck. In July 1966, Richard Speck brutally murdered eight student nurses in their townhouse in Chicago, Illinois. One resident of the townhouse, Corazon Amurao, rolled under a bed and was not killed. She gave a description of the murderer to the police, including the fact that he had a tattoo on his left forearm that read "Born to raise hell." Two days later Richard Speck attempted suicide and was taken to Cook County Hospital. A physician who treated him noticed the distinctive tattoo and the resemblance to the composite sketch printed in the newspaper and called the police. Speck was arrested and subsequently convicted. Others, of course, may have observed this man's face and forearm; but they did not have his name and address. This information was crucial, and the physician acquired it in his role as a medical professional. It seems, then, that the physician breached confidence, but nobody thought that he did wrong.

Another example of breaching confidence to protect the public interest concerns a more recent case. In 1980 in Wyckoff, New Jersey, Donald Chapman dragged a twenty-three-year-old woman into a woods and tied her to a tree.[8] Several hours later he returned and committed what a judge called a "barbarous" act of rape, torture, and murder, using such instruments as a shovel, a pickax, scissors, and razors. Having served a twelve-year prison term, Chapman returned to Wyckoff in November 1992. Days before his release, Kay Jackson, a psychologist who treated him in prison, warned a prosecutor that Chapman still fantasized about young women and had vowed to rape again. This information was passed on to local police, and on Chapman's release they conducted an around-the-clock surveillance of his home, at a cost of $2,000 a day. Psychologist Jackson breached confidence, but few protests were heard. There may be significant moral differences between this case and that of Richard Speck, but Jackson's rationale was to protect innocent people from harm.

Other examples abound, and we shall discuss some of these later. More importantly, we shall examine the moral legitimacy of each of these three types of exceptions and ask whether each is morally defensible.

Confidentiality: The Moral Issues

To begin investigating confidentiality from the moral point of view, we need to ask why confidentiality is morally important. More specifically, we need to ask what reasons might be given to support the claim that the confidentiality obligation for health care professionals is absolute. Here two arguments will be examined; one is deontological and the other is consequentialist.[9]

The first argument for the confidentiality obligation is deontological. It appeals to the idea that health care practitioners tacitly promise to keep information about patients confidential and it is based on the right to privacy. One way of putting the argument is this:

1. There is a presumption, an implied understanding, that communications between patients and health care practitioners are private.

2. As a result of this presumption, patients reveal things to health care practitioners that they would not reveal otherwise.

3. A patient's right to privacy gives him the right to control who has access to this information.

4. So, health care professionals violate a patient's right to privacy if they give information about that patient to others without that patient's consent.

The principle of autonomy underlies this argument, for that principle is at the root of the right to privacy. Autonomy refers to freedom and self-control, and the right to privacy concerns controlling who has access to certain information about oneself. The sociological background is crucial to this argument. In Western societies, at least, there is a wide presumption that the communications with health care workers are confidential. Thus information is acquired under that guise. Without this presumption, privacy would not be at stake unless patients *explicitly solicited* a promise of confidentiality before entering into a professional relationship with physicians. But in our society, that action is regarded as unnecessary, precisely because there is an implied promise.

A second argument for the confidentiality obligation is based on a consequentialist principle. The underlying idea is that health care practitioners cannot do their jobs properly unless the confidentiality obligation is absolute.[10] To show this point, we begin by assuming the opposite and showing what the likely consequences will be:

1. Suppose that there are exceptions to the confidentiality obligation.

2. If patients recognize that there are exceptions to the confidentiality obligation, this will adversely affect their willingness to divulge information to health care professionals.

3. Patients will be inclined to hide potentially embarrassing information for fear that it will be divulged to others.

4. In some cases, potential patients will forgo treatment altogether because of the fear of embarrassment, or worse.

5. But unless ill persons seek treatment and provide health care professionals with all of the information they have about their condition, health care professionals cannot do their jobs properly.

6. So, unless the confidentiality obligation is absolute, health care professionals cannot do their jobs properly.

This argument appeals to what is best for ill persons as a class. They need to seek medical treatment and be encouraged to be forthright with health care workers so that they will receive accurate diagnoses and the most suitable treatment possible. But they will be so encouraged only if they are assured that information they give to health care providers will not be divulged to others.

This same sort of consequentialist argument is used to establish a confidentiality obligation in other professions too. Thus, one may argue that for attorneys to be able to protect their clients' legal rights, those clients must be completely forthcoming with attorneys. But they will be forthcoming only if they are assured that what they tell their attorneys is strictly confidential. Similar arguments are used to show that confidentiality must prevail in communications between clergy and those to whom they minister, between journalists and their sources, and between counselors and clients.

These two arguments are rooted in the fundamental values discussed in Chapter 1: autonomy and well-being. The deontological argument says that without confidentiality, health care practitioners fail to respect their patients' autonomy. The consequentialist argument says that the job of health care workers is to protect and promote the well-being of patients, which cannot be accomplished without confidentiality. Together the arguments make a very strong case for confidentiality.

Still, we might wonder whether the confidentiality obligation is absolute. Cases such as those of Richard Speck and Donald Chapman lead many to doubt that it is. Here we shall critically examine in detail the three exceptions to the confidentiality rule endorsed by the AMA, two of which were also endorsed by the BMA. In each of the three cases we shall ask whether the proposed exception should be approved. We can envision the task this way. If we were trying to develop an ideal rule for health care practitioners regarding confidentiality, which exceptions, if any, would we include?

To prevent misunderstandings, let us emphasize that the AMA's three exceptions specify circumstances under which physicians are *permitted* to breach a patient's confidence; they do *not* say that physicians are *required* to do so. Presumably these are matters of judgment. Let us now consider the three exceptions.

Breaching Confidence When It Is in the Interest of the Individual Patient If a patient is not competent, then either health care practitioners will have to reveal information about that patient to others, usually family members, or will have to make all treatment decisions themselves. The more challenging case concerns competent patients.[11] We have to envision cases in which patients are competent, but physicians judge that those patients would be better off if others (usually family members) had certain information about their medical condition. As noted earlier, examples include patients whom physicians believe may attempt suicide and likely noncompliant patients. This exception is based on paternalism, and even if the particular examples seem persuasive, there may be doubts about how broadly the exception can be applied.

These doubts come to the fore when we examine the well-known case of Robert Browne.[12] Browne was a family physician in England. In 1971, a clinic in Birmingham, England, sent a report to Browne indicating that they had prescribed an oral contraceptive for one of his patients, a teenager, Miss X. The clinic routinely issued such reports to patients' family physicians unless the patients forbade them to do so. Browne was also the physician to Miss X's parents. Soon after he received this report, Miss X's father came to Browne for a visit. Browne asked Mr. X whether his daughter had married recently. When he learned that she had not, he told the father that his daughter was taking birth control pills. Browne's actions created an uproar, and he was charged with unprofessional conduct. However, at a hearing before the British General Medical Council, Browne appealed to one of the exceptions to the confidentiality rule endorsed by the BMA. He said that he breached confidence to protect the patient's own interests. He pointed to what he called the physical, psychological, and moral hazards of the pill. Among other things, he professed to be protecting Miss X from a sense of guilt that she might experience were she to take the pill without consulting her parents.

The Disciplinary Committee of the British General Medical Council did not find Browne guilty of professional misconduct. They recognized that the clause that allowed physicians to breach confidence if they judged that it was in the patient's best interests gave physicians considerable leeway, and they could not say that Browne was being insincere in his application of this clause. They also recognized, however, that changes in the code were needed. The exception in question basically gave physicians a blank check, which was too much power. The BMA, therefore, amended their statement on confidentiality in 1971. They dropped the exception to which Browne had appealed and replaced it with a statement far less paternalistic.

The amended clause says that if a physician believes that it is in a patient's medical interests to have confidential information disclosed to a third party, then the physician has a duty to try to convince the patient to allow this information to be disclosed to that person; but if the patient refuses to allow that information to be divulged, that refusal must be respected. This approach puts the burden on physicians to explain to patients why it is in their interests that someone else have certain information. When patients consent, it is no breach of confidence.

Unless some qualification is placed on this exception, physicians are given a blank check to breach confidence on paternalistic grounds. And with that, there is no way to block actions such as those of Browne. The change instituted by the BMA seems wise, therefore, and this first exception, unless qualified, is unjustifiable. Put more accurately, breaching confidence for paternalistic reasons is justified only when patients are not competent. But when patients are competent, their consent should be obtained before a third party is given information about them for their own good.

Breaching Confidence When Required by Law   A second exception endorsed by the AMA says that physicians are justified in breaching confidence if required by law to do so. This means that physicians are justified in breaching confidence *simply because* the law requires them to do so.

In raising doubts about the legitimacy of this exception, we may begin with a mundane observation.[13] Laws are made by legislators, and they can and sometimes do enact legislation that is morally unjustified. Consider an extreme *hypothetical* example. Suppose that a law were passed requiring physicians to report to a federal agency any patient testing positive for HIV. The purpose of the legislation is to develop a registry of persons with HIV and make it available to insurance companies and prospective employers. Such legislation is morally questionable, and physicians should consider refusing to comply with it. Given this, why might anyone think that physicians are warranted in breaching confidence simply because they are required by law to do so? At least two reasons can be cited to justify this second exception in spite of the fact that there can be bad laws.

The first reason to justify this AMA exception points to the serious effects on society of disobeying the law. Robert Veatch articulates this reasoning eloquently:

> The physician, after all, is a citizen of the land and subject to the laws of the land. To decide to break the law, even when it appears justified by a professional code of ethics with a principle as well established as that of confidentiality, is no trivial decision; it is civil disobedience.
>   . . . But to reject legal authority routinely and without due thought is anarchistic. No society could survive the indiscriminate personal acceptance or rejection of law. If the physician is to avoid considering himself different from other citizens, he must treat civil disobedience with appropriate seriousness.[14]

The argument, then, is that to break the law is to engage in an act of civil disobedience. But no society can survive if its citizens disobey the law indiscriminately.

This is a familiar contention and often advanced in contexts much broader than the one of concern here. The argument is unconvincing, however; it is based on an exaggeration. Isolated acts of civil disobedience by physicians will not constitute rejecting legal authority "routinely" and will not destroy society's fabric; if societies were that delicate, most would long ago have ceased to exist. After all, illegal acts occur frequently. Moreover, those who deny that physicians are justified in breaching confidence merely because the law requires that they do so are not advocating *indiscriminate* disobedience. The occasions for questioning the law will presumably be rare.

There is an additional problem with this argument. Even if it were not based on an exaggeration, it would not show that physicians are justified in breaching confidence when the law requires them to do so. Instead, it would only show that society is justified, on the basis of self-defense, in punishing physicians who refuse to breach confidence when demanded by law.[15] But this observation should not shock us, because there is no guarantee that the demands of the law and those of morality will always be in harmony, which leads naturally to the next point.

The second reason in support of this exception to the confidentiality rule begins with the observation that anyone who openly disobeys the law will be punished, by either fine or incarceration. Thus, to disobey the law is to incur a great sacrifice. But no one is morally required to make great sacrifices. Such acts are called *supererogatory*, acts above and beyond the call of duty. Since agents are permitted to refrain from performing supererogatory acts, physicians are justified in breaching confidence when required by law; to deny this is to confuse acts that are required with those that are beyond the call of duty.

This argument in defense of the second exception is also flawed, however. It is based on the false assumption that morality never requires agents to make great sacrifices. Journalists plausibly regard themselves as required to endure incarceration rather than to reveal confidential sources. And parents are often obliged to undergo severe hardships for their children's welfare. To assume that all self-sacrificial acts are supererogatory is simply incorrect; some are morally required. It is reasonable to expect that members of a helping profession, such as medicine, will be among those who are sometimes obligated to make such sacrifices. And indeed many health care providers do regard themselves as being so obligated. Timothy Quill cites a well-known case in which he puts himself at legal risk to assure that one of his patients has a comfortable death.[16]

There may, of course, be other reasons to support the exception under discussion here, and if so, they must be addressed. But even if there are no such reasons, it is important to understand that it *does not follow* that physicians ought to disregard the law when it demands that they breach confidence. Instead, the conclusion to draw is that they should examine each law on its own merits. If the law is morally sound, they may be justified in breaching confidence; if it is not morally sound, they must consider disobedience. Indeed, one might reasonably think that all citizens have a comparable responsibility.

Those who endorse breaching confidence because required by law are probably impressed with the particular statutes with which they are acquainted, such as requirements to report gunshot wounds, infectious diseases, and evidence of child abuse. But arguably there is a common justification for these laws: each is necessary to protect the public interest. A gunshot wound suggests likelihood of foul play and is evidence that the welfare of others may be endangered; thus, investigation is warranted. Similarly, steps must be taken to arrest infectious diseases to minimize harm and prevent epidemics. And when evidence of child abuse is found, there is reason to believe that the well-being of vulnerable minors is threatened and an immediate investigation is called for. In any particular case, the goal is to see that justice is done. But ultimately these considerations are rule utilitarian and suggest that these laws are morally sound.

The upshot of this discussion is that this second exception is also not justified. It is important to realize, however, that these criticisms do not deny that each citizen has an obligation to obey duly enacted laws. The point instead is that physicians also have an obligation to keep information about their patients confidential. The obligations of confidentiality and obedience to the law can, in certain circumstances, conflict. Those who claim that physicians may breach confidentiality whenever required by law to do so are saying that the obligation to obey the law is *always* more important than and takes precedence over the obligation of confidentiality. But such a position is too simplistic. The strength of the general obligation to obey the law is context-dependent and cannot be divorced from a particular statute's content. The obligation to obey a morally justifiable law is stronger than the obligation to obey a law that is unjustifiable, and the former are more likely to prevail in cases of conflict than are the latter.

Breaching Confidence to Protect the Public Interest The cases of Richard Speck and Donald Chapman discussed earlier are instances of breaching confidence to protect innocent people from harm. There are many other cases like this. One concerns a bus driver in New York during the 1960s.[17] This man's doctor told him that he had a bad heart and cautioned him not to drive. The bus driver refused to tell his company about the heart condition for fear he would lose his job. The physician did not breach confidence, and the worst-case scenario played out. Thirty people were killed when the driver had a heart attack and plunged his bus into the East River. Some were critical of the physician, claiming that he should have breached confidence to protect the welfare of innocent people.

Laws requiring health care practitioners to report contagious diseases, evidence of child abuse, and gunshot wounds seem to be based on this same principle: these laws are designed to protect the public interest.

This exception, then, seems correct; health care professionals are justified in breaching confidence when doing so is necessary to protect others from harm. Complications arise, however, when one tries to *apply* this exception to particular cases. It is sometimes difficult to determine whether breaching confidence prevents more harm than it causes. This difficulty will be illustrated by discussing the well-known case of Tatiana Tarasoff.[18]

Tatiana Tarasoff and Prosenjit Poddar, students at the University of California at Berkeley, had been dating in 1969. They had different perceptions about the nature of their relationship. Poddar regarded it as quite serious; Tarasoff, as casual. When Tarasoff ended the relationship, Poddar became depressed. He went to Lawrence Moore, a psychologist at the university, for therapy. In August 1969, Poddar told Moore that he wanted to kill his former girlfriend when she returned to the country. Tarasoff was visiting in Brazil during that summer. Though Poddar did not mention Tarasoff's name, Moore could have easily determined her identity. Moore decided that Poddar should be committed to a mental hospital for observation. He sent a letter to the campus police asking for their help in securing Poddar's confinement. Poddar was taken into custody, but the police decided that he was rational and released him because he promised to stay away from Tarasoff. When the police informed Moore about Poddar's release, Moore's superior, Harvey Powelson, ordered that no further action be taken. On October 27, 1969, Poddar killed Tarasoff.

Tarasoff's parents brought suit against the university regents, the campus police, and Moore and Powelson. They argued that the doctors and the police had an obligation to warn them or their daughter about Poddar's threats. The Supreme Court of California, in a split decision issued in 1976, ruled that a doctor does have a duty to warn third parties if a mentally ill patient threatens to harm them. The author of the majority opinion, Justice Mathew Tobriner, argued that the public safety outweighs the importance of confidentiality and that the "protective privilege ends where the public peril begins." Justice William Clark, in a dissenting opinion, argued that confidentiality between psychotherapists and patients should be maintained in such cases.

Justice Clark might seem opposed to breaching confidence to protect the public interest. But a careful reading of his dissenting opinion suggests something different. Justice Clark argues that if psychotherapists breach confidence in cases of this sort, such action will actually cause more harm than it prevents; and many involved in psychotherapy and counseling agree. What sort of reasoning is offered to support this position? Defenders of the minority position claim that far more patients express desires to commit acts of violence than actually carry them out. In addition, they claim that psychologists and psychiatrists are very poor at predicting which patients, among those who express such desires, will actually act on them. As a result, if psychotherapists must issue warnings in all of these cases, there will be many breachings, most of which were unnecessary. And if breaching confidence becomes common, either patients will withhold information from their therapists, or they will cease treatment altogether. But if that outcome happens, many individuals who could have been helped will not be, and the likely result is even more acts of violence.

It is important not to misunderstand this argument. The factual claim that psychotherapists cannot predict accurately what patients will carry out threats to commit acts of violence is crucial. For if that claim is true, then essentially therapists must either report all such threats or none at all, since they have no reliable basis for further distinguishing among them. But this tactic will result in so many breaches of confidence that the cumulative effects will be negative. The reasoning here is rule utilitarian (as explained in Chapter 1).

Many factual claims underlie the minority position, and until those can be adequately assessed, it is hard to resolve this debate. For example, the minority position assumes that psychotherapy is effective in preventing some patients from committing acts of violence. It also assumes that effective treatment requires that patients communicate honestly with therapists. These assumptions may be true, but they should be recognized as assumptions.

Another crucial assumption is that the practice of breaching confidence will deter patients from being honest or seeking help at all. While the relevant empirical studies have only just begun, some preliminary data support this crucial assumption. The state of Maryland passed a law in 1989 requiring therapists to report any patient who admits to sexually abusing a child. When the law was first considered, opponents argued that patients would avoid therapy if they knew that they would be reported. One study suggests that this effect is exactly what is happening.[19] Before this law was passed, an average of seven abusers a year voluntarily entered the Johns Hopkins Sexual Disorders Clinic for treatment. And every year approximately twenty-one patients already in therapy would admit that they had sexually abused a child. Since the law went into effect, the number of admitted sexual abusers of children dropped to zero. If subsequent empirical studies point in the same direction, such data will lend some credence to the minority view in the Tarasoff case.

One other case of this sort is worth mentioning briefly. This occurred in Texas in 1966. A Dallas psychiatrist let it be known, after the fact, that one of his patients, Charles Whitman, had expressed fantasies about shooting people. And in fact, about two weeks after Richard Speck's killings, Whitman ascended a tower on the campus of the University of Texas and began shooting people. He was only stopped when a police sharp-shooter killed him. Whitman's psychiatrist did not warn anyone about the threats. But one major difference is apparent between the Whitman and Tarasoff cases: Whitman did not identify specific persons whom he intended to harm. There really was no individual whom Whitman's psychiatrist could have warned. Unless the psychiatrist thought that Whitman could be involuntarily confined on grounds of danger to self or others, there was nothing that he could do. An interesting question is whether the ability to predict acts of violence varies depending on whether a specific victim is identified.

To reiterate, the point being made about the Tarasoff case is not to oppose breaching confidence to protect others from harm. Rather, the point is that breaching confidence itself is likely to cause some harm because of its adverse effects on the patient–health care practitioner relationship. As a result, *applying* this exception to particular cases is difficult. And in some cases breaching confidence may cause more harm than it prevents.

Breaching the Confidence of One Patient to Protect Another Patient Patient consequentialism urges health care professionals always to do what is best for their patients. But as we noted in Chapter 1, one problem with this view is that the interests of two patients may conflict. The issue of confidentiality provides an illustration of this point.

Breaching the confidence of one patient to protect a second patient need not be regarded as a separate exception; it may be looked at as a special instance of protecting others from harm. But it does make the situation more difficult for health care providers because it puts them in a position of facing conflicting loyalties, as a well-known case will make clear.

David, age twenty-one, had a troubled past, including conflicts with his father.[20] David gained exemption from the draft when his physician attested to the fact that David was homosexual. Five years later, Joan visited her family physician for a premarital serological exam. It was the same physician who had treated David. Joan, twenty-four, had been under this physician's care for a number of years. They had a warm relationship, and so it was natural for the physician to ask about Joan's fiancé. When he did, he learned that she was going to marry David. She said that she had not known David long, but was sure of her choice. The physician said nothing. David and Joan were married shortly thereafter. They separated after six months, and the marriage was annulled on the basis of nonconsummation. Joan learned that she and David had shared the same physician and that the physician had known that David was homosexual. Joan suffered depression as a result of this experience and was angry with her physician for not telling her about David's homosexuality. She felt that she could have been spared much emotional trauma and that her physician was responsible for not acting. Joan felt that her family physician should be concerned with her overall well-being, including her emotional health.

A physician who must choose between two patients is caught in a difficult moral problem. Joan's physician might have tried strategies to minimize the difficulties. He might, for example, have called David and suggested that he be honest with Joan. That might not have worked, however; David might have just said no. And some may question a physician calling a former patient. He might also have engaged Joan in a conversation and asked her whether she was sure about her choice. But it would have been difficult to do this without either being intrusive or telling her what he knew about David. While we need not try to resolve this case here, many have said that there are just too many uncertainties involved to warrant the physician breaching confidence. For all the physician knew, David may have been bisexual, thus not precluding ordinary marital relations. Or David may have changed, as some say. Perhaps most importantly, however, family physicians are not experts at predicting what factors contribute to the success or failure of a marriage. Perhaps no one has expertise here!

In this case, from the doctor's perspective, the claim that breaching confidence will prevent significant harm is speculative at best. The confidentiality obligation is firm enough that it should be breached only when one can be confident that doing so prevents significant harm to others. Still, cases may occur in which physicians can prevent significant harm to one of their patients only by breaching the confidence of a second patient.

Suppose that a physician diagnoses a man as HIV-positive and tells him that he must inform his wife about this and alter his sexual practices.

The man says that he will not inform his wife and will not change his sexual practices. The wife is also a patient of this physician. Here the likelihood that significant harm will occur is great, and, if it has not already occurred, the chances that the physician can prevent it are good.

Both deontological and consequentialist considerations show that the confidentiality obligation is strong. And while we are not warranted in saying that breaching confidence to prevent significant harm to others is the only legitimate exception to the confidentiality rule, it is the one easiest to defend.

TRUTH TELLING

There is an obligation to be truthful in communications with others. Lying or intentionally deceiving another is usually wrong. And, in some contexts, withholding the truth may be just as bad. The principal focus of this section will be on whether health care practitioners are ever justified in lying to patients about their own medical condition—especially about their diagnosis and prognosis—or withholding the truth from patients. Here we consider only obligations regarding competent patients. In many cases, it may be clear that when patients lack the capacity to make their own decisions, at least withholding the truth from them is justified. Physician Sherwin Nuland describes a case in which a patient's doctor and wife decide to withhold from him that he has Alzheimer's disease because he lacks the ability to comprehend the implications of such a diagnosis.[21] It should be acknowledged, however, that judgments about whether patients have the capacity to make their own decisions are sometimes difficult to make.

Most codes of medical ethics make statements about confidentiality. By contrast, these same codes are typically silent about the obligation, if any, to be truthful with patients about their condition. One notable exception is "A Patient's Bill of Rights" (issued by the American Hospital Association in 1973). The second clause of this document says:

> The patient has a right to obtain from his physician complete current information concerning his diagnosis, treatment, and prognosis in terms the patient can be reasonably expected to understand. When it is not medically advisable to give such information to the patient, the information should be made available to an appropriate person in his behalf.

This statement affirms that patients have a right to complete and accurate information regarding their diagnosis and prognosis, and it even specifies that this information must be conveyed in terms that patients can understand. The statement allows for an exception, however. If it is not "medically advisable" to give the patient this information, then it should be made available to a close associate of the patient—presumably a spouse, parent, child, or sibling. Nothing is said about when it might be medically inadvisable to disclose complete information to the patient. Apparently that judgment is to be made by physicians on a case-by-case basis.

If sociological surveys are accurate, the attitudes and practices of physicians regarding being truthful with patients about a diagnosis of terminal illness have changed radically.[22] In a 1961 survey, 88 percent of physicians who responded said that their usual policy was not to tell patients when the diagnosis was cancer. During this same time, several surveys of patients were done, and 80 to 90 percent said that they wanted to know the truth if they had cancer. We do not know whether the physicians' actions were in accord with their responses to the surveys, nor do we know whether what the patients said matches what they would really have wanted. But the disparity here was so great that we must conclude that at this time, physicians and patients were operating with different moral beliefs in this area. Perhaps there has always been such a disparity, for more than two centuries ago, Samuel Johnson said:

> I deny the lawfulness of telling a lie to a sick man for fear of alarming him. You have no business with consequences; you are to tell the truth. Besides, you are not sure what effects your telling him that he is in danger may have. It may bring his distemper to a crisis, and that may cure him. Of all lying, I have the greatest abhorrence of this, because I believe it has been frequently practised on myself.[23]

In 1979, a group of researchers asked physicians almost identical questions that were posed in the 1961 survey. The results were dramatically different. This time 98 percent of the physicians who responded reported that their usual policy was to tell cancer patients the truth about their diagnosis and prognosis. Such a shift is remarkable. In part, this reversal probably constitutes a genuine moral change. There is little doubt that during this time medical paternalism came under attack and patient autonomy was emphasized. But other factors probably contributed to this change too.[24] Rates of survival from some forms of cancer improved. More treatment options were available to patients. And social attitudes toward persons with cancer changed; the stigma once associated with the disease had begun to fade.

Here we shall examine the issue of being truthful with patients, looking at both arguments that support the older view—the paternalistic withholding of the truth—and those that support the change. It should be noted at the outset that some maintain that there is a morally important difference between lying and merely withholding the truth; they say that while the former may be prohibited, the latter is not.[25] This point may be true in some contexts, but it seems doubtful in the field of medicine, at least when patients are competent, partly because of patients' expectations (as will be explained later). In any case, positive arguments given here will suggest that an obligation of honesty is incompatible with both lying and withholding the truth; thus, this distinction is not emphasized here.

Arguments about Truth Telling

Physicians who supported deceiving patients in particular cases probably reacted in part against a kind of deontological absolutism. According to this view, people have a duty to tell the truth, period, and no exceptions are allowed. And some think that in medical contexts, withholding the truth from patients about their own condition can be just as wrong as directly lying. Perhaps this is the view that was being articulated by Samuel Johnson in the passage cited earlier. The eighteenth-century German philosopher Immanuel Kant seems committed to the same position, as the following passage shows:

> The duty of being truthful . . . is unconditional. . . . Although in telling a certain lie I do not actually do anyone a wrong, I formally but not materially violate the principle of right. . . . To be truthful (honest) in all declarations, therefore, is a sacred and absolutely commanding decree of reason, limited by no expediency.[26]

Kant, it seems, allows for no exceptions to the truth-telling rule. This stance is the kind of position that physicians and other health care practitioners encountered and reacted against. Doctors would sometimes say that this view is nothing but "truth for truth's sake." As such, this is just name calling, but an important criticism underlies the slogan.

Any credible deontological system will affirm several moral values, and honesty in communications will be one of those. But other rules and values are important, too, among which is the obligation to prevent harm or suffering when one can do so. These rules and values can, on occasion, conflict, which shows that not all can be absolute. The rule regarding truth telling can conflict with the rule about preventing harm, such as when the crazed husband intent on doing harm asks you whether you know the whereabouts of his wife. In this case, most think that lying is permissible. This suggests that the absolutist position against lying is mistaken. In medical contexts, if being truthful with patients about their condition will cause them to suffer, then the health care practitioner will face this same conflict. And even if how best to resolve the conflict is not always obvious, this case still shows that deontological absolutism is questionable, for it assumes either that truth telling is the only important moral value or that it always takes precedence over any value with which it conflicts.

Consequentialist Case for Withholding the Truth   Thirty years ago, it was apparently common for physicians to withhold the diagnosis of terminal illness from their patients. Undoubtedly the reason most did so was fear of the consequences of being truthful. As the quote from Johnson says, at the very least they feared alarming the sick person. Their motivation was to do what was best for patients, and they believed that sometimes lying to patients (or at least withholding the truth) was what was best.[27] Such a position may be based on patient consequentialism, and the underlying argument is this:

1. **Health care practitioners should always do what will, on balance, most benefit (or least harm) their patients.**
2. **In some cases, withholding the truth from patients about their own condition is what will most benefit those patients.**
3. **So, in those cases health care practitioners should withhold the truth from patients about their own condition.**

This argument does not recommend always deceiving patients; rather, situations should be handled on a case-by-case basis. The first premise of this argument states the principle of patient consequentialism. It directs health care providers always to do what is best for patients. The second premise says that in some situations some patients will be better off if they are not told the truth about their own condition. But why is this so? Why affirm premise 2? When defenders of this argument claim that telling the patients the truth about their own condition can harm them, they usually have in mind the cases in which the diagnosis is terminal illness. If certain patients are given this information, bad consequences are likely to ensue. Some patients will experience great anxiety, and as a result their last days will be very unpleasant. Some patients will give up hope and lose the will to live, thus dying sooner than they otherwise would have. Some patients may commit suicide. Sometimes errors in diagnoses are made, and when patients are erroneously told that they are terminally ill, they will have been caused needless suffering.[28] And even when the diagnosis is correct, sometimes patients recover miraculously;

when that occurs, again patients have been caused needless suffering. In addition, some say that because of scientific complexities, patients cannot be told the "whole truth"; they cannot understand it, and they have gross misconceptions about illnesses.[29]

According to this position, the judgment of whether to be truthful with patients is context-dependent. No doubt in most situations health care professionals should be truthful with patients about their own condition, especially when the news is not bad. But in some cases, being truthful will be bad for the patient. This is probably the idea being conveyed in "A Patient's Bill of Rights" when it says that it is sometimes "not medically advisable" to tell patients the truth about their own diagnoses and prognoses. This consequentialist argument, then, seems to be the foundation for the "old-time" view that deceiving patients is sometimes permissible.

Consequentialist Case for Always Telling the Truth You might think that anyone who endorses consequentialism will be forced to say that withholding the truth from patients about their own condition is sometimes the right thing to do. This is not the case, however. There is a consequentialist argument for always telling patients the truth about their own diagnoses and prognoses[30] that begins with the same premise as the previous argument:

1. **Health care practitioners should always do what will, on balance, most benefit (or least harm) their patients.**
2. **Withholding the truth from patients about their own condition will, as a policy, cause more harm than being honest with them.**
3. **So, health care practitioners should adopt the policy of being honest with patients about their own condition.**

Premise 1 states the patient consequentialist principle of counseling health care providers always to do what is best for patients. As we saw, this approach can allow for much paternalism. But this argument says that if health care workers want to do what is best for patients, they will be truthful with patients. Obviously the key to understanding this argument concerns the explanation of premise 2.

The defenders of this argument claim that many bad consequences for patients will ensue if health care professionals withhold the truth from patients about their own prognoses and diagnoses. They make several points. First, those who defend withholding the truth from patients usually do not advocate telling bald lies, such as "You're just fine." Instead, they avoid the truth and say things like, "We need to do further tests." If that approach is taken, it is likely to heighten patient anxiety. Not knowing the truth and being left to wonder can cause as much suffering as hearing bad news.

Second, even when patients have terminal illnesses, sometimes treatments exist that will extend their lives by months and make their last days more pleasant. If patients are to take these treatments seriously, they must know the gravity of their situation.

Third, there are personal and economic decisions that patients cannot make responsibly unless they are fully informed about their own condition. If you knew that you only had a few months to live, you would probably want to spend that time with your loved ones. But if you are not given the pertinent information, you are deprived of exercising this option. And the financial decisions that people make are likely to vary greatly if they know that they are terminally ill. Such persons are unlikely to make speculative investments and may reasonably choose not to accept expensive treatment that merely delays death. What this third point shows is that a person's best interests are not reducible merely to medical interests. The consequentialist argument for withholding the truth focuses only on medical interests, but that is not all that patients care about.

A fourth point in support of premise 2 concerns the issue of trying to predict how patients will respond to bad news. Physicians are not experts at predicting how patients will respond to the news that they have a serious illness.[31] Perhaps no one has expertise in this area. That may have been Samuel Johnson's point when he said to physicians, "You have no business with consequences." If physicians are not good at predicting who might respond poorly to bad news, then unless most patients react in this way physicians have no good basis for lying.

Finally, an important long-range consequence is associated with dishonesty: patients will lose faith in physicians. One recent small-scale study conducted in a hospital setting examined the use of deception by nurses.[32] The results suggest that deception can have adverse effects on trust between patients and nurses. Indeed, one might suspect that the practice of lying to prevent anxiety and mental anguish will be self-defeating. Patients will reasonably judge that even if they have a terminal illness, their physician will not be truthful about this. Suppose that you have had chronic headaches. You fear that you have a malignant brain tumor. You go to your physician. If physicians routinely lie to patients about these matters, then you already know what your physician is going to tell you; she will say that you do not have a malignant tumor. Because you know of the deceitful practice common in the profession, this gives you no comfort. And even if in fact you do not have a malignant tumor, the physician cannot give you comfort, for you believe that that is what the doctor tells everyone. Thus, the practice of deceit, if widespread, undermines its own purpose. It makes health care practitioners unable to give comfort even when there is good reason for it.

This consequentialist argument for being truthful with patients about their condition does not appeal to patients' rights. This argument focuses only on beneficence and is compatible with the paternalistic model. It says, essentially, that if health care professionals are concerned to do only what is best for their patients, they should be truthful with them.

How can there be two consequentialist arguments, each beginning with the same major premise, that yield opposite conclusions? Part of the answer is that the consequentialist argument for withholding the truth focuses only on *certain medical* interests of patients—namely, extending the length of survival—while the consequentialist argument for telling the truth tries to take into account other patient interests that are affected by medical decisions. But there is another important difference. The consequentialist argument for withholding the truth from patients urges health care professionals to address this issue on a case-by-case basis. This point leads one to think, quite reasonably, that what is good for Jack may not be good for Jill. Defenders of the consequentialist argument for telling patients the truth claim that this perspective is short-sighted. Handling situations on a case-by-case basis is itself a policy that has ramifications beyond those particular cases. Lying to Jack will affect later cases, at least when the general populace becomes aware of how these cases are handled. So, one must compare on consequentialist grounds the policy of always being honest with patients with the policy of lying when doing so would seem to be best for that particular patient. And those who favor honesty say that the overall consequences of adopting the policy of being truthful are better than the overall consequences of adopting the policy of deceiving patients in certain cases. The point is that the consequences are better for patients themselves.

Contractual Argument for Being Truthful The consequentialist argument for being truthful makes no reference to the rights of patients and says nothing about the importance of autonomy; this feature is in contrast with the contractual argument.[33] One way of understanding the contractual argument is this:

1. The contractual model is the correct way to understand the relationship between patients and health care practitioners.
2. According to the contractual model, patients are to make or approve all major decisions because they have the right to self-determination.

3. But patients cannot exercise their right to self-determination in medical contexts unless they have complete and accurate information about their own condition.

4. So, health care practitioners have an obligation to provide patients with complete and accurate information about their condition.

According to the contractual argument, there is a presumption that patients will receive from health care practitioners any potentially useful information about their own condition so that they can make informed decisions. Obviously a patient's diagnosis and prognosis constitute potentially useful information to that patient. So, health care professionals incur an obligation to provide patients with that information. Of course, if the diagnosis and prognosis are poor, this information should be conveyed in a kind, sensitive manner; but nevertheless it should be conveyed. To do less is to fail to meet one's obligations and violate the patient's right to self-determination.

Taken together, the consequentialist and contractual arguments make a very strong case for being truthful with patients about their own condition. They establish a strong prima facie obligation of honesty. It is important to realize, however, that these are very different arguments. The consequentialist argument appeals to beneficence and says nothing about patients' rights, such as the right to self-determination. This argument is compatible with the paternalistic model. The contractual argument appeals to the rights of patients and is not compatible with the paternalistic model. The fact that the same conclusion can be supported from such radically different perspectives is impressive, which gives health care providers multiple reasons for being truthful. But one still wonders whether there are any exceptions.

Possible Exceptions to the Truth-Telling Rule

It does not follow from all of this that the obligation to be truthful with patients is absolute. While many possible exceptions might be considered, here we shall discuss four.

Withholding the Truth from a Patient at the Family's Request The scene is familiar enough. The patient is a male in his forties.[34] He had a stroke and before that had been bothered by headaches and nausea. He is admitted to the neurological center of a teaching hospital. Surgery is performed, and a malignant brain tumor is discovered. As the patient is recovering from surgery, the physician approaches his wife. He tells her about the grim findings and indicates that her husband has at best five months to live. The woman is initially stunned but quickly takes charge. She tells the neurosurgeon in no uncertain terms that her husband should not be told about the tumor. According to the wife, he has a history of denying reality and handles bad news poorly. The physician wonders whether he should honor the wife's request.

We might ask initially why it is tempting to endorse this exception and comply with the woman's request. Two things stand out. First, we may assume that the family knows the patient better and longer than anyone else. Given this intimate knowledge, the family is better able than health care providers to determine how the patient will respond and whether the patient can handle bad news. Second, we may assume that the family cares about the patient and wants what will best promote the patient's interests. Those who both know a person well and want what is best for that person are in a good position to look out for his interests.

In spite of these considerations, there are reasons to doubt the appropriateness of withholding the truth from a patient simply because the family says to do so. First, no matter how it is described, complying with the family's wishes involves treating the patient paternalistically. This violates the patient's right to self-determination.

Second, the family may not know the patient best. People often underestimate their loved ones. Perhaps it is natural to see those whom one loves the most as vulnerable and wish to protect them. In some cases, outsiders have a more objective perspective and see that the patient is stronger than the family thinks. Cases have been reported in which the patient and the family both know the truth, and each asks the physician not to tell the other. Perhaps love sometimes distorts vision.

Third, the family may not always want what is best for the patient. It is natural to assume that the family is loving, and perhaps in most cases they are. But assuming that this is always the case would be naive. To cite just one possibility, family members may believe that the patient is considering writing a new will excluding them and that news of his terminal illness will prompt him to act. We hope that these cases are rare, but we cannot assume that they never occur.

Fourth, the patient may suspect the truth and want to talk about it with family members. But a conspiracy of silence will make it difficult for the patient to initiate appropriate conversations.

Finally, there is something very troubling about this case. The physician has communicated to the family about the patient's condition before telling the patient. This behavior is an unacceptable breach of confidence unless previously authorized by the patient.[35] Of course, family members want to know that the patient survived the surgery, and telling them that news is permissible. To give them a detailed account of the findings without the patient's prior consent, however, is not proper. Here conversations should occur before the surgery. Perhaps most patients will consent to having details conveyed to family members before they themselves receive the information. But the conversations should occur first.

The bulk of the weight suggests that this exception is not legitimate; withholding the truth from patients at the request of the family is not justified without additional argumentation.

Withholding the Truth at the Patient's Own Request Again the scene is familiar. The patient has had persistent pain in his hips.[36] Thoughts that it was a pulled muscle were refuted by the duration and increase in severity of the pain. One physician thought that it was arthritis, but medication effective for pain resulting from that affliction was inefficacious. Finally, the patient made an appointment with an orthopedic surgeon. The patient did not give voice to his real fear—that he had bone cancer. When he met with the orthopedic surgeon, his message was clear: he wanted the surgeon to do whatever was medically necessary, but he did not want to be bothered with the details. The patient did not want to hear the word *cancer*. Should the physician abide by the patient's request?

One way to look at this case is that the patient has, in effect, contracted into a paternalistic relationship. Since the patient has expressed his wishes while competent, complying with them is not a case of unacceptable paternalism. Although this attitude places an enormous burden on a physician, if both parties are agreeable, then perhaps there is no moral problem.

There is, however, a second way to view this case. Something is troubling about the patient's request itself. This patient has a wife and three children. One who has such responsibilities may not have a right not to know the truth about his own medical condition. After all, knowledge that one is terminally ill may alter greatly the sort of personal and economic decisions that one will make. For example, this man would surely not make high-risk investments or drop his life insurance policy if he knew that death were imminent. Given this man's obligations, one can argue that he is being irresponsible in requesting that he not be told the truth about his condition. But for the physician, the issue is whether to comply with the request. One position holds that the physician's only obligations are to this patient; so, if this is what the patient really wants and the physician is willing to accept this burden, then going along with his request is permissible. The other position says that it is wrong for physicians to assist patients in behavior designed to avoid moral responsibilities. According to this view, the physician should refuse at the outset and make it clear to the patient why he is doing so. One supporting this position might point to cases like those of Richard Speck and Donald Chapman to refute the claim that physicians' only obligations are to their patients.

Beauchamp and Childress describe a troubling case that falls under this category.[37] A thirty-five-year-old man in a high-risk group for AIDS went to a physician because of symptoms consistent with infection with HIV. He consented to be tested for HIV. However, on the day that the physician received the test results but before she had conveyed them to the patient, the patient telephoned to say that he wanted to cancel the test; he did not want the results. As it turned out, this patient was infected with HIV. The physician decided to inform him of the results. She felt that he should know this to reduce the risks to others with whom he had intimate contact; his attempt to avoid this information was irresponsible and dangerous to others. It is perhaps not clear whether complying with this patient's request and not giving him the test results would constitute "assisting" him in his irresponsible behavior. But this physician, at least, thought that she had an obligation to give the patient information that he should not have avoided.

We should note that cultural differences among societies can complicate this issue. Physician Antonella Surbone describes problems she encountered after being trained in the United States and then returning to Italy to practice.[38] In the United States she was taught to respect autonomy and tell patients the truth. But in Italy, she reports, families and physicians often shield patients from painful truths. Indeed, this approach seems to be expected by all. And apparently this is true in many other countries.[39]

In an interesting way, this cultural context combines these first two exceptions because the family may be claiming that the patient himself does not want to be told the truth. Benjamin Freedman suggests a novel way of handling such cases.[40] He recommends that such patients be offered the truth. Health care providers can tell these patients that they are very ill and then ask them whether they understand, whether they have any questions, and whether they want to talk. Patients who do not respond to these cues apparently do not want to know more. In such a context, this second exception takes on a different look.

Deceiving Patients for the Good of Others   Suppose that you found yourself in a situation where the following conditions were true: (1) By deceiving another person you could obtain significant benefits for others. (2) Your deceit carries with it no risk or harm to the person. (3) The benefits for others can be obtained only if you deceive this person.

Judging from past practice, people in the field of medicine seem to have believed that they were in such a situation when it came to providing training for medical students.[41] Apparently it was once common for third- and fourth-year medical students to administer treatment to patients in teaching hospitals without those patients knowing that they were being treated by students. Sometimes patients called them "doctor" and were not corrected. The justification for this deception was based on an argument like that in the previous paragraph. It was claimed that medical students must get on-the-job training if they are to be prepared to practice medicine; this practice benefits all of society. Patients in teaching hospitals are not harmed by this because the students are administering routine treatment that is highly supervised. But the deception is necessary because too many patients would irrationally refuse to permit the students to treat them if they were fully informed. This argument is utilitarian.

Most of us would not want to be on the receiving end of this sort of deception. It is a case of manipulation and violates the right to self-determination. Though this practice is less prevalent now, it is still an issue.[42] It is more common, however, for patients who enter teaching hospitals to be told that medical students are part of the health care team; these patients must give consent before the students can administer any treatment to them. No evidence suggests that medical students are not receiving adequate training. Apparently enough patients give consent. If so, this situation suggests either that people's attitudes have changed greatly, that they are more trusting of the medical profession and students, or that the medical establishment underestimated people in assuming that they would refuse to allow students to be involved in their treatment. If it really were true that medical students could not get adequate training without this deceptive practice, we would have a very difficult problem. For we would have to choose between sacrificing a valuable utilitarian end or compromising the rights of patients. Such choices are troubling. For now we seem able to achieve the end without employing the dubious means.

Withholding the Truth to Avoid Disastrous Consequences Even with both consequentialist and deontological arguments supporting an obligation to be truthful with competent patients, one wonders whether there are not extreme cases where that obligation is defeated by more important moral considerations. Cases can be produced that give even the strongest advocates of honesty cause for pause.

Consider the following example.[43] A serious automobile accident occurs. Among those involved are a woman and her five-year-old daughter. The mother is seriously injured, and the daughter is killed instantly. The woman suffered internal injuries and needs surgery. She is rushed to the hospital. As she is being prepared for surgery, she regains consciousness and asks the nurses about the condition of her daughter. They believe that if she is told the truth at this time, it will have adverse effects on her—she might lose the will to live or go into shock, and her chances of surviving the operation will be diminished. This situation calls for an immediate decision; it leaves no time for moral reflection. Based on the likely consequences, the nurses tell the woman that her daughter was taken to another hospital, and they do not know about her condition. The woman survives the surgery and only then is told the truth.

This is a persuasive case. Few are inclined to say that the nurses made the wrong decision. But if that decision leads to endorsing this general exception—withholding the truth to avoid disastrous consequences—it creates a problem. It would seem that health care practitioners could cite this same exception to justify withholding the truth from some terminally ill patients about their own condition. Put another way, this exception seems to embrace the principle underlying the consequentialist argument for withholding the truth. So how can we endorse this exception without being led back to the "old-time" view?

If it is the example itself that leads some to endorse the exception, then we might look for relevant differences between it and cases of withholding the truth from terminally ill persons. Two differences stand out. First, in the example the health care professionals plan to withhold the truth from the patient only temporarily. Once she recovers, then of course she will be fully informed. Second, the example is not a case of withholding the truth from a patient about her own condition. Instead, she is being deceived about the condition of someone else. While some may dispute the relevance of this second point, the idea is that deceiving someone about her own condition is more paternalistic, or at least more objectionable, than temporarily deceiving her about someone else's condition. If this argument is convincing, then perhaps this exception can be cast in such a way as to preclude allowing health care workers to withhold the truth from patients about their own condition.

We conclude this section with two cases in which some will be tempted to deceive patients about their own condition or treatment. First, consider the patient who is addicted to pain-killing medication.[44] Members of the health care team believe that the patient can be comfortable without the medication, so they decide to wean him from the drug by gradually diluting the dosage. In effect, the patient is given a placebo without his knowledge. They believe that this strategy will be successful only if deceit is employed.

The second case is more unusual. The patient is a seventeen-year-old student at a local high school. She is a cheerleader and honors student.

She and her parents had initially come to the physician because she had yet to begin having menstrual periods. Now the physician has scheduled a conference with the patient and parents about his findings. What this physician has discovered is that his patient is not biologically female; "she" is a male. Karotyping, a process of analyzing the chromosomes of a cell, revealed an xy rather than xx alignment. The patient is a victim of testicular feminization, a disorder in which a genetically male child appears from birth to be female. Because of tissue unresponsiveness to male hormones, the testicles fail to descend during pregnancy. At birth, the infant looks like a female. The patient has a shallow vagina but of course no uterus. Due to hormonal abnormalities, there is usually no facial hair. The diagnosis is usually made during an investigation of amenorrhea, as in this case. Should this physician tell a seventeen-year-old who has been raised as a female that "she" is really a male? Should he tell the parents and let them decide? Certainly this person needs to be told that "she" is sterile. And because of a high risk of cancer, the abdominal gonads need to be removed. But what exactly should the physician tell the patient? And how? These are some of the difficulties that arise when discussing this fourth possible exception to the rule about truth telling.

A CONFLICT BETWEEN CONFIDENTIALITY AND HONESTY

A five-year-old girl has been a patient for three years with renal failure secondary to glomerulonephritis.[45] She has been on dialysis, but renal transplantation is being considered. Whether it will be effective is not known, but attempting it is preferable to subjecting this patient to long-term dialysis. The results of tissue typing indicate that the patient will be difficult to match. Her brother and sister are too young to serve as donors. Tests show that the mother is not histocompatible. The girl's father then undergoes tests, and the results reveal that he is compatible and could serve as a donor. The nephrologist informs the father of these results. He also tells the father that the girl's prognosis is uncertain and that the transplant might not work, though it seems to be her best chance. After some reflection, the father decides not to donate a kidney to his daughter; he admits that he is afraid. However, he does not want his family to know that he has refused to donate. He fears that they will think that he is a coward and blame him for any of his daughter's subsequent medical problems. If the nephrologist tells the family the truth about the father, it will ruin his family life, he believes. Therefore, he asks the physician to tell the family that he is not histocompatible. The physician agrees to tell the family that the father should not donate a kidney for medical reasons.

This nephrologist appears to be caught in a serious moral problem. It appears that he either has to deceive the family or breach the confidence of the father; he chose not to breach confidence. In thinking about this case, several points should be taken into account. First, when the physician told the family that the father should not donate for medical reasons, he probably was not lying. Candidates to serve as living kidney donors are usually tested for emotional as well as physical fitness. One reason for this practice is that living kidney donors often experience depression after the organ is removed. So it may well be true that the father was not a medically suitable donor. Of course, the family did not interpret what the nephrologist said in this way; they no doubt took him to mean that the father was not histocompatible.

Second, the nephrologist is not withholding information from a patient about his own condition. This point is a little complicated, however; for while his immediate patient is the five-year-old girl, in another sense he is treating the entire family. At least, they seemed to have approached this as a family matter. Unfortunately, unbeknownst to all of the other parties, the father was not an enthusiastic participant.

Third, if the physician had chosen to breach confidence, presumably his reason would have been to maximize the chances that the girl would receive a kidney. Because she is difficult to match, he knows that the chances of finding a suitable nonrelated donor are very slim. So, he might have reasoned, "If I tell the rest of the family the truth, they will put pressure on the father and he will consent." The nephrologist did *not* employ this strategy, which may be a good thing. Predicting how the father and the family will react if all know the truth is a very tricky matter. Such a strategy could just as easily have backfired. The father may have remained adamant, and the marriage may have dissolved. And, to make a point similar to one in the case of David and Joan earlier, it seems clear that nephrologists are not experts at predicting how families will respond to this kind of information. Maybe no one has expertise in this area of family dynamics; certainly there is no special reason to think that nephrologists do.

SUMMARY

Three models of the health care practitioner–patient relationship were discussed. The engineering model appropriately emphasizes patient autonomy but implausibly does not allow health care providers to use their own moral judgments when they practice medicine. The paternalistic model properly stresses beneficence, urging health professionals to do what is best for patients, but it gives no weight to the autonomous wishes of patients. The contractual model, which respects the autonomy of both parties, directs practitioners to make recommendations based on beneficence; but patients may not be compelled to accept these recommendations, nor may providers be forced to act against their own values. When, for reasons such as unconsciousness, age, or mental disability, patients cannot make their own medical decisions, the paternalistic model seems best. But when patients have the capacity to make decisions, the contractual model seems more suitable, because it alone accords appropriate weight to the autonomy of both patients and practitioners. Determining when patients have the capacity to make their own decisions is not always easy, however; in many cases, the contractual model may be an ideal that cannot be attained.

The confidentiality obligation can be supported by both consequentialist and deontological concerns. That and historical considerations make a strong case for this moral requirement. Nevertheless, the obligation may not be absolute. Three possible exceptions to the confidentiality obligation, endorsed by the AMA and others, are breaching confidence to promote the patient's own interests, breaching confidence because required by law to do so, and breaching confidence to protect the public interest. The case for the first two of these exceptions is weak. And though the third exception seems legitimate, applying it in actual cases can be difficult.

The obligation to be truthful with patients about their own diagnoses and prognoses too can be supported by both consequentialist and deontological considerations. Yet, again, one wonders whether there are any exceptions. The most likely candidates here are withholding the truth from a patient at the family's request, withholding the truth from a patient at that patient's own request, deceiving patients for the good of others, and withholding the truth to avoid disastrous consequences.

Suggestions for Further Reading

Adams, Jean. "Confidentiality and Huntington's Chorea." *Journal of Medical Ethics*, Vol. 16 (1990), pp. 196–199.

Beauchamp, Tom L., and James F. Childress. *Principles of Biomedical Ethics*, 4th ed. (New York: Oxford University Press, 1994), Chapter 7.

Berlin, F. S., H. M. Malin, and S. Dean. "Effects of Statutes Requiring Psychiatrists to Report Suspected Sexual Abuse of Children." *American Journal of Psychiatry*, Vol. 148 (1991), pp. 449–453.

Boyd, Kenneth M. "HIV Infection and AIDS: The Ethics of Medical Confidentiality." *Journal of Medical Ethics*, Vol. 18 (1992), pp. 173–179.

Buchanan, Allen. "Medical Paternalism." *Philosophy and Public Affairs*, Vol. 7 (1978), pp. 370–390.

Ellin, Joseph S. "Lying and Deception: The Solution to a Dilemma in Medical Ethics." In Thomas A. Mappes and Jane S. Zembaty (eds.), *Biomedical Ethics*, 3d ed. (New York: McGraw-Hill, 1991), pp. 81–87.

Freedman, Benjamin. "Offering Truth." *The Archives of Internal Medicine*, Vol. 153 (1993), pp. 572–576.

Jackson, Jennifer. "Telling the Truth." *Journal of Medical Ethics*, Vol. 17 (1991), pp. 5–9.

McConnell, Terrance. "Confidentiality and the Law." *Journal of Medical Ethics*, Vol. 20 (1994), pp. 47–49.

Teasdale, Kevin, and Gerry Kent. "The Use of Deception in Nursing." *Journal of Medical Ethics*, Vol. 21 (1995), pp. 77–81.

Veatch, Robert M. *Case Studies in Medical Ethics* (Cambridge, MA: Harvard University Press, 1977), Chapters 5 and 6.

Veatch, Robert M. *Death, Dying, and the Biological Revolution*, rev. ed. (New Haven, CT: Yale University Press, 1989), Chapter 7.

Veatch, Robert M. "Models for Ethical Medicine in a Revolutionary Age." In Thomas A. Mappes and Jane S. Zembaty (eds.), *Biomedical Ethics*, 3d ed. (New York: McGraw-Hill, 1991), pp. 55–58.

Walter, LeRoy. "The Principle of Medical Confidentiality." In Thomas A. Mappes and Jane S. Zembaty (eds.), *Biomedical Ethics*, 3d ed. (New York: McGraw-Hill, 1991), pp. 162–165.

Winslade, William J. "Confidentiality." In Warren T. Reich (ed.), *Encyclopedia of Bioethics*, rev. ed. (Upper Saddle River, NJ: Prentice Hall, 1995), Vol. 1, pp. 451–459.

Notes

1. Robert M. Veatch, "Models for Ethical Medicine in a Revolutionary Age," in Thomas A. Mappes and Jane S. Zembaty (eds.), *Biomedical Ethics*, 3d ed. (New York: McGraw-Hill, 1991), pp. 55–58. (Veatch's essay was originally published in *The Hastings Center Report*, Vol. 2 [June 1972].) Veatch actually discusses four models. The *collegial* model is not explained here.

2. Veatch, "Models for Ethical Medicine in a Revolutionary Age," p. 56.

3. Physician Timothy E. Quill, clearly committed to a model of shared decision making in medicine, describes a case in which he initially disagreed with a

request of one of his patients but later decided to grant her wishes. See *Death and Dignity* (New York: Norton, 1993), pp. 9–18, 45–48.

4. The various codes of medical ethics referred to here are reprinted in the appendix.

5. See Robert M. Veatch, *Case Studies in Medical Ethics* (Cambridge, MA: Harvard University Press, 1977), pp. 117–118, 131–135.

6. See Veatch, *Case Studies in Medical Ethics*, pp. 117, 355.

7. On this topic, see editorials in the *Archives of Psychiatric Nursing*, Vol. VI (October 1992), pp. 255–256, and Vol. VII (June 1993), pp. 123–124.

8. For an account of this case, see the *Greensboro News and Record*, February 9, 1993.

9. Versions of these arguments are discussed in LeRoy Walters, "The Principle of Medical Confidentiality," in Thomas A. Mappes and Jane S. Zembaty (eds.), *Biomedical Ethics*, 3d ed. (New York: McGraw-Hill, 1991), pp. 162–165.

10. Some think that no consequentialist argument can be given in support of absolute obligations (or society's enforcing an obligation as absolute). But this belief is mistaken. To understand why, see Rolf E. Sartorius, *Individual Conduct and Social Norms* (Belmont, CA: Dickenson, 1975).

11. Throughout this book, *competent* is used to designate patients who have the capacity to make their own medical decisions, and *incompetent* designates patients who lack that capacity. See Allen Buchanan and Dan Brock, *Deciding for Others: The Ethics of Surrogate Decision Making* (New York: Cambridge University Press, 1989), Chapter 1.

12. See Veatch, *Case Studies in Medical Ethics*, pp. 131–135.

13. Most of the material in this section is borrowed from my "Confidentiality and the Law," *Journal of Medical Ethics*, Vol. 20 (1994), pp. 47–49. It is used here with permission of the BMJ Publishing Group.

14. Veatch, *Case Studies in Medical Ethics*, pp. 126–127.

15. Veatch, *Case Studies in Medical Ethics*, p. 127. Veatch may concur with this since he concludes that physicians must treat civil disobedience "with appropriate seriousness."

16. See Quill, *Death and Dignity*, pp. 9–25.

17. This case is discussed in Walters, "The Principle of Medical Confidentiality," p. 164.

18. See Justice Mathew O. Tobriner, "Majority Opinion in *Tarasoff v. Regents of the University of California*," and Justice William P. Clark, "Dissenting Opinion in *Tarasoff v. Regents of the University of California*," in Mappes and Zembaty (eds.), *Biomedical Ethics*, pp. 165–173. See also, Tom L. Beauchamp and James F. Childress, *Principles of Biomedical Ethics*, 4th ed. (New York: Oxford University Press, 1994), pp. 509–512.

19. F. S. Berlin, H. M. Malin, and S. Dean, "Effects of Statutes Requiring Psychiatrists to Report Suspected Sexual Abuse of Children," *American Journal of Psychiatry*, Vol. 148 (1991), pp. 449–453.

20. This case is presented in *Hastings Center Report*, Vol. 7 (1977), p. 15.

21. Sherwin B. Nuland, *How We Die* (New York: Knopf, 1994), pp. 95ff.

22. See Donald Oken, "What to Tell Cancer Patients: A Study of Medical Attitudes," *Journal of the American Medical Association*, Vol. 175 (1961), pp. 1120–1128, and Dennis H. Novack, Robin Plumer, Raymond Smith, Herbert Ochitil, Gary Morrow, and John Bennett, "Changes in Physicians' Attitudes Toward Telling the Cancer Patient," *Journal of the American Medical Association*, Vol. 241 (1979), pp. 897–900. For a detailed discussion of these and other relevant surveys, see Robert M. Veatch, *Death, Dying, and the Biological Revolution*, rev. ed. (New Haven, CT: Yale University Press, 1989), pp. 182–185. See also Beauchamp and Childress, *Principles of Biomedical Ethics*, pp. 398–399.

23. Quoted in Alan Donagan, *The Theory of Morality* (Chicago: University of Chicago Press, 1977), p. 89.

24. On this point, see Beauchamp and Childress, *Principles of Biomedical Ethics*, p. 398.

25. See, e.g., Joseph S. Ellin, "Lying and Deception: The Solution to a Dilemma in Medical Ethics," in Mappes and Zembaty (eds.), *Biomedical Ethics*, pp. 81–87.

26. Immanuel Kant, "On the Supposed Right to Tell Lies from Benevolent Motives," in Thomas K. Abbott (trans.), *Kant's Critique of Practical Reason and Other Works on the Theory of Ethics* (London: Longmans, Green, 1909), pp. 361–365.

27. This position is discussed in Veatch, *Death, Dying, and the Biological Revolution*, pp. 167–169.

28. For a case of this sort, see Oliver M. Cope, "Man, Mind, and Medicine," in Samuel Gorovitz, Ruth Macklin, Andrew Jameton, John O'Connor, and Susan Sherwin (eds.), *Moral Problems in Medicine*, 2d ed. (Upper Saddle River, NJ: Prentice Hall, 1983), pp. 222–223.

29. These points are made by Mack Lipkin, "On Lying to Patients," *Newsweek*, June 4, 1979, p. 13. Here Lipkin defends a version of the consequentialist argument for withholding the truth from patients. (Note that this is as late as 1979.)

30. This argument is discussed in Veatch, *Death, Dying, and the Biological Revolution*, pp. 171–175.

31. See Allen Buchanan, "Medical Paternalism," *Philosophy and Public Affairs*, Vol. 7 (1978), pp. 379ff.

32. Kevin Teasdale and Gerry Kent, "The Use of Deception in Nursing," *Journal of Medical Ethics*, Vol. 21 (1995), pp. 77–81.

33. A version of the contractual argument is discussed in Veatch, *Death, Dying, and the Biological Revolution*, pp. 175–177.

34. A case of this sort is discussed in Veatch, *Case Studies in Medical Ethics*, pp. 153–154.

35. For a similar point, see Beauchamp and Childress, *Principles of Biomedical Ethics*, pp. 398–399. See also *Guidelines on the Termination of Life-Sustaining Treat-*

ment and the Care of the Dying (Bloomington: Indiana University Press, 1987), p. 22.

36. A case of this sort is presented in Veatch, *Case Studies in Medical Ethics,* pp. 154–155.

37. Beauchamp and Childress, *Principles of Biomedical Ethics,* p. 403.

38. Antonella Surbone, "Truth Telling to the Patient," *Journal of the American Medical Association,* Vol. 268 (1992), pp. 1661–1662.

39. P. Dalla-Vorgia, K. Katsouyanni, T. Garanis, G. Touloumi, P. Drogari, and A. Koutselinis, "Attitudes of a Mediterranean Population to the Truth-Telling Issue," *Journal of Medical Ethics,* Vol. 18 (1992), pp. 67–74.

40. Benjamin Freedman, "Offering Truth," *Archives of Internal Medicine,* Vol. 153 (1993), pp. 572–576.

41. See Veatch, *Case Studies in Medical Ethics,* pp. 147–149.

42. See Jay E. Kantor, *Medical Ethics for Physicians-in-Training* (New York: Plenum Medical, 1989), pp. 67–73.

43. This case is presented in Joseph S. Ellin, "Lying and Deception: The Solution to a Dilemma in Medical Ethics," in Mappes and Zembaty (eds.), *Biomedical Ethics,* pp. 86–87. Ellin attributes this case to Bernard Gert and Charles Culver. A similar case was related to me many years ago by Cynthia Pickles, who encountered it in her experience as a nurse.

44. For a discussion of cases of this sort, see Ellin, "Lying and Deception," pp. 82–83, and Veatch, *Case Studies in Medical Ethics,* pp. 151–153.

45. This case is presented in Melvin D. Levine, Lee Scott, and William J. Curran, "Ethics Rounds in a Children's Medical Center," *Pediatrics,* Vol. 60 (1977), p. 205.

CHAPTER 3

Treatment and Informed Consent

WHEN, IF EVER, is it morally appropriate to administer treatment to a patient without that patient's consent? This issue arises most compellingly when a patient refuses lifesaving treatment for reasons that health care practitioners think are poor. This topic, more directly than any other, forces us to confront questions about paternalism. Of course, in Chapter 2 we saw that one reason that some cite for breaching a patient's confidence is to protect that patient's own well-being; we also saw that the classic argument for withholding the truth from patients about their own medical condition is rooted in paternalism. But here the issue is raised more dramatically, for several reasons. First, refusal of treatment can lead to immediate harm, so the good to be promoted by paternalistic intervention is obvious. Second, actually imposing treatment on patients without their consent is a physically intrusive act, far more so than is typically the case when confidentiality is breached or the truth is withheld from patients.

The issue of treatment without consent also involves a direct conflict between two basic principles. The principle of autonomy suggests that competent patients have the right to refuse treatment if they wish. But the principle of beneficence instructs health care professionals to protect the well-being of patients, which may require administering treatment in spite of their wishes to the contrary. In such cases, one of these principles must yield.

LIBERTY-LIMITING PRINCIPLES

Our general concern here is to understand the conditions under which one person may restrict the freedom of another.[1] We assume what is called the *liberty principle*: any interference with liberty or restriction of a person's freedom requires justification. This principle affirms our commitment to autonomy. It does not deny that we are sometimes justified in restricting another's freedom. But it says that the burden of proof is on those who propose to interfere with the behavior of another. Since groups and institutions, as well as individuals, can restrict the freedom of persons, the liberty principle puts a burden of proof on them too. Thus, when the state passes laws, it restricts the freedom of its citizens, so justification for the laws is needed.

Even though any interference with a person's freedom requires justification, it is widely believed that some principles do provide such warrant. The most obvious and justifiable reason for restricting a person's freedom is stated in the *harm principle*: we may restrict a person's freedom to prevent that person from harming other nonconsenting parties. This principle says, in effect, that as a society we are justified in enforcing the principle of nonmaleficence. Any civilized society will endorse this principle.

Three points of clarification about the harm principle should be made. First, it allows a society to prevent a person from harming *others*. But it does not apply to self-inflicted harm; that sort is covered by a different principle, paternalism. Second, it only allows society to prevent harm inflicted on *nonconsenting* parties. If two or more consenting adults are inflicting harm on each other—as in the sport of boxing—the harm principle would not justify restricting that behavior. Again, that would be covered by paternalism. Finally, the harm principle is usually understood to apply to both *private* and *public* harm. Private harm is harm perpetrated against specific nonconsenting individuals. Examples of behavior prohibited on the basis of the private harm principle include killing, stealing, and assault. Public harm is harm done to institutions or systems that promote the public interest. Tax evasion, contempt of court, defamation of public property, and desertion from the military are examples of behavior that is adverse to the public interest without typically harming any specific identifiable individual. For the most part, our concern will be with private harm.

While there are many questions about the proper formulation and application of the harm principle,[2] here we shall assume that it is a legitimate liberty-limiting principle. Indeed, one might argue that society's enforcing the harm principle maximizes individual liberty. Enforcing the harm principle does restrict individual freedom; it prevents a person from harming others. But it also protects a person from harm that might be inflicted by others. Given that each individual has to live with others, this is a good trade. Each gives up some freedom but in return gains something, namely, protection against harm perpetrated by others.

Other liberty-limiting principles are more controversial. For the purpose of discussing the issues surrounding treatment and informed consent, the most important principle is paternalism. According to *paternalism*, we may force a person to do something or do something to a person without consent for that person's own good. Both institutions and individuals can treat a person paternalistically. Laws designed to prevent or discourage people from harming themselves illustrate institutional paternalism. Examples include laws requiring drivers to wear seat belts, laws compelling motorcyclists to wear helmets, and laws prohibiting people from swimming on public beaches without lifeguards. Examples of one individual treating another paternalistically include a parent preventing her child from crossing a busy street alone and a physician administering lifesaving treatment to a patient against that patient's wishes.

During the past few decades, medical paternalism has been widely criticized. But most people recognize that a blanket prohibition against paternalism is too simplistic, for some instances of paternalism seem proper (such as preventing a child from crossing a dangerous street alone) while others do not (such as forcing an adult to stop consuming fattening food). These points suggest that further distinctions are needed.

Philosophers usually distinguish between two forms of paternalism, weak and strong.[3] According to *weak paternalism*, we may do something to a person without his consent and for his own good only when that person's conduct is substantially nonvoluntary or when temporary intervention is necessary to determine whether the conduct is nonvoluntary. Among the things that render conduct nonvoluntary are ignorance, serious mental defect, inner compulsion, and coercion. Since these factors can vary in degree, whether conduct is voluntary or nonvoluntary is a matter of degree.

The idea underlying weak paternalism is this. To the extent that behavior is nonvoluntary, it does not represent the agent's autonomous choices; in one sense, it is not the agent's own. So if an agent's nonvoluntary behavior puts him at risk, it is not the agent's autonomous choice. If in such cases others interfere with the agent's behavior for the agent's own good, they are exhibiting beneficence. But their beneficence does not conflict with the agent's autonomy, because the agent's behavior is not autonomously chosen. Stopping the young child from crossing the busy street alone is weakly paternalistic. And involuntarily committing a person who has a serious psychiatric disorder and is a danger to himself is weakly paternalistic.

John Stuart Mill, a nineteenth-century British philosopher otherwise opposed to paternalism, gives an example of justified weak paternalism.[4] Mill asks us to imagine a case in which a man is about to cross an unsafe bridge. If the man does so, he is likely to plunge to his death. Mill says that we are justified in preventing the man from crossing the bridge to determine whether he realizes that the bridge is unsafe. Though Mill himself does not fill in the details for this case, presumably if the man said that he fully understood the danger, Mill would oppose detaining him further. The purpose of the intervention is to determine whether his risky behavior is substantially voluntary; if it is, further restriction is not warranted.

Strong paternalism says that we may do something to a person without consent for her own good even when that person's behavior is substantially voluntary. Like all paternalism, strong paternalism is based on the principle of beneficence. But unlike weak paternalism, strong paternalism allows beneficence to take precedence over autonomy in cases of conflict. If we prevented competent adults from participating in automobile races simply because of the risks to themselves, that would be strongly paternalistic. If a physician imposed lifesaving medical treatment on a competent patient against that patient's wishes, that too would be strongly paternalistic.

Weak paternalism is easier to justify than strong paternalism because only strong paternalism involves interfering with an agent's autonomous choices. And though there is a genuine distinction between weak and strong paternalism, in some cases determining whether intervention for the agent's own good is weakly or strongly paternalistic is difficult. Suppose that a nineteen-year-old woman is diagnosed with anorexia nervosa. She will not eat because she fears becoming obese. Even when she loses weight, she still claims to feel fat. Are her family and health care professionals justified in force-feeding her? Her behavior is no doubt not fully voluntary, but is it *substantially* nonvoluntary? Or imagine that a patient has an irrational fear of a certain treatment. Suppose, for example, that a twenty-one-year-old male has a fear of needles and as a result refuses a needed medical treatment. Is his choice substantially nonvoluntary? Borderline cases like these make the topic of justified paternalism very difficult.

TREATMENT WITHOUT CONSENT: THE LEGAL STATUS

Concerning the legal right to refuse medical treatment, two distinctions are important. One is the distinction between treatment administered in situations in which patients can consent to or refuse the treatment and treatment in emergency situations in which patients are unable to consent or refuse. The other distinction is between a competent patient who refuses treatment and a legal guardian who refuses treatment for an incompetent patient.

Emergency Situations

The law is simplest and most straightforward regarding the treatment of persons in emergencies. If a person is incapable of expressing consent or refusal, if treatment is needed immediately, and if no one is available who is authorized to speak for that person, then physicians may administer treatment. Consent is assumed. Physicians are given the therapeutic privilege of assuming that in these situations patients want what is medically best for them. Even if it should turn out that the patient has serious objections to the form of treatment that was administered (for example, it turns out that the patient is a Jehovah's Witness and the treatment was a blood transfusion), no law has been broken and the physician is not liable, assuming that the form of treatment is standard and the physician is not guilty of negligence. The rationale underlying this aspect of our legal system is weak paternalism. Patients in emergency situations are not capable of giving either consent or refusal; so in doing what is medically best for them, health care providers are not unjustifiably interfering with their autonomy. They are practicing beneficence, but not at the expense of autonomy.

Though physicians are *permitted* to administer treatment in emergency situations, matters may be more complicated, depending on the status of Good Samaritan legislation in a physician's state. All states have *minimal* Good Samaritan legislation, the object of which is to protect health care professionals from legal liability if they administer treatment in emergency situations. Some states may go beyond this, however, and *require* medical professionals to provide assistance in such emergencies.

One other complication is worth mentioning. Paramedics and emergency medical teams may sometimes be called to assist the same patient on several occasions during the same night. The patient may be conscious and competent the first few occasions and refuse any intervention. Later, however, that patient may be unconscious. It may not be entirely clear how this should be handled, but typically emergency medical teams regard each call as new and so give needed treatment when the patient is not competent.

Competent Patients

What is the legal situation when competent patients refuse medical treatment? May physicians overrule patients' wishes and administer needed therapy? In the United States, the type of case that has arisen most frequently here is when a patient refuses treatment for religious reasons. In these cases the courts appeal to the principle of autonomy and a patient's right to self-determination. In effect, this approach involves a rejection of strong paternalism. Numerous cases have affirmed that a competent adult's refusal of medical treatment must be honored. As early as 1914, in a New York case, Justice Cardoza ruled that "every human being of adult years and sound mind has a right to determine what shall be done with his own body."[5] And in 1960, ruling on a case in which a blood transfusion had been given to a patient against his will, the Kansas Supreme Court said:

> Anglo-American law starts with the premise of thoroughgoing self-determination. It follows that each man is considered master of his own body, and he may, if he be of sound mind, expressly prohibit the performance of lifesaving surgery, or other medical treatment. A doctor might well believe that an operation or form of treatment is desirable or necessary but the law does not permit him to substitute his own judgment for that of the patient by any form of artifice or deception.[6]

Most of the court cases in which this issue has arisen have involved Jehovah's Witnesses who have refused blood transfusions even though their physicians have warned them that they are necessary to save their lives. Jehovah's Witnesses believe that blood transfusions are forbidden by God's law. They point to certain passages in the Bible (Genesis 9: 3–4, Leviticus 17: 10–14, Deuteronomy 12: 33, and Acts 15: 28–29), passages that proscribe "blood eating," to support their belief.[7] If you assume, as Jehovah's Witnesses do, that there is a God, that God's law forbids blood transfusions, and that the penalty for violating that law is eternal damnation, then you would have to agree that the position of the Jehovah's Witness is entirely rational. Apparently, however, since most people are willing to undergo blood transfusions if medically necessary, most do not accept all of those assumptions. Given this, it might be tempting to force Jehovah's Witnesses to undergo the treatment for their own good. Such an action would be strongly paternalistic. In defense of it, some might argue that Jehovah's Witnesses are attaching irrational weights to the various values in question. This attitude would provide health care practitioners with a rationale to interfere and promote the patients' medical well-being.

But in spite of the fact that most people disagree with Jehovah's Witnesses about the permissibility of blood transfusions, most oppose violating their religious freedom. In cases like this, it is wrong to force treatment on competent adults, even when the treatment in question is lifesaving. This position probably evolved because we will go to great lengths to allow people to make their own moral and religious decisions. When possible, we tolerate evaluative differences. We should not be unclear here, however. A person's reason for refusing medical treatment need not be religious; a person has a right to refuse medical treatment for *any reason*, and normally that refusal must be respected. In 1962, a New York court put it this way:

> It is the individual who is the subject of a medical decision who has the final say and this must necessarily be so in a system of government which gives the greatest possible protection to the individual in the furtherance of his own desires.[8]

The courts have consistently ruled, then, that competent individuals may refuse medical treatment on religious grounds or for any other reason. Not only that, but physicians who administer treatment against the wishes of a competent patient may be guilty of battery.

This situation does not mean that people may do anything in the name of religion. In general, the state may not interfere with a person's religious *beliefs*, nor may it do anything to try to alter such beliefs. But if a religious *practice*—actions based on religious beliefs—threatens to harm innocent persons, the state may impose restrictions. Thus, it is permissible for states to require school attendance, to require that parochial schools satisfy certain minimal standards, and to require that children be immunized against certain diseases. These requirements are justified by the harm principle and appropriate even if parents have religious objections. This is not to say that the state does not go beyond the harm principle when it restricts religious practices. States forbid polygamy, and some proscribe the use of poisonous snakes in religious ceremonies even if only consenting adults are present, and it is not obvious that either of these prohibitions is based on preventing harm to nonconsenting parties. As noted earlier, in allowing competent persons to refuse lifesaving medical treatment, states in effect reject strong paternalism. Yet, in other areas states seem to endorse strong paternalism, such as when they require the use of seat belts and the use of helmets by cyclists. Such oddities are perhaps to be expected.

Guardians and Incompetent Patients

For legal purposes, any individual under eighteen years old is presumed not competent to make medical decisions. In some circumstances, however, this presumption can be rebutted.[9] One such case concerns so-called *emancipated minors*. A person under the age of eighteen may petition the court for full rights as an adult. This grant of adult status is based on the minor's maturity and needs. Circumstances that typically qualify a minor to consent to medical treatment include marriage and service in the military. Special medical conditions constitute a second type of situation in which minors may consent to medical care without parental authorization. These include but are not limited to abuse, communicable diseases, alcohol and drug use, and pregnancy. The idea here is that if parental consent were required for treatment of these conditions, it might discourage minors from seeking needed care.

Let us now consider situations in which the patient is presumed incompetent, the presumption is not rebutted, but someone is available who is authorized to speak for the patient, such as a spouse, parent, or guardian. When a patient is incompetent, that person is not capable of making his own medical decisions. The notion of competence is relative to the task at hand; a person may be competent to do some things and not competent to do others.[10] So understood, competence is a legal notion. Suppose that a guardian (a general term used to designate the person authorized to speak for the patient) refuses recommended treatment for an incompetent patient. Must this refusal be honored? In discussing this question, we must distinguish two types of cases: when the refused treatment is necessary to save the patient's life and when the treatment is desirable but not necessary to save the patient's life. Discussion of the first type of case will be somewhat extensive.

The courts have ruled in a number of cases in which guardians (usually parents) have refused lifesaving treatment for incompetents (usually children). Two similar cases occurred in 1952, in Illinois and Missouri.[11] In each of these cases, an infant was suffering from Rh incompatibility, erythroblastosis fetalis. This problem occurs when the blood from an Rh-positive fetus seeps into the Rh-negative mother's circulatory system, and it is at least the second such pregnancy. In such situations, Rh antibodies will be produced in the maternal blood and may cross the placenta into the fetal circulation. This condition can result in the infant's death, so a blood transfusion is needed at birth. In the cases in question, however, the parents were Jehovah's Witnesses and refused to give their consent for the transfusions. The courts, in each of these cases, declared the infant a "neglected dependent" and appointed a guardian to give consent for the needed treatment.

In cases of this sort, hospitals obviously must act quickly. Action is typically done by telephoning a judge and securing the needed order. The courts have said that while parents have a right to refuse lifesaving treatment for themselves, they do not have a right to make martyrs of their children. In these cases, the freedom of parents to engage in certain religious *practices* is being limited. While parents normally have the right to make decisions regarding their children, they are not free to endanger the children's lives. The basis for this restriction is the harm principle. Parents can harm their children through neglect. Not providing adequate food or shelter would typically be considered neglect, and so too is refusing lifesaving medical treatment.

A well-known case that illustrates the underlying principles here is that of Delores Heston.[12] This case occurred in New Jersey in 1971. Heston was a twenty-two-year-old Jehovah's Witness who was severely injured in an automobile accident. Among other things, she had a ruptured spleen. When she entered the hospital, she was in shock and, in the judgment of the health care practitioners, incoherent. She was temporarily incompetent. Her injuries were such that surgery needed to be performed and blood administered. The medical team sought the consent of her mother, also a Jehovah's Witness, but she refused. Mrs. Heston even signed a release of liability for the hospital. But the hospital applied to a judge to have a guardian appointed. The court complied with this request, surgery was performed, blood was administered, and Heston's life was saved. We noted earlier that courts allow competent adults to refuse medical treatment even if that results in death. The decision in the case of Delores Heston is entirely consistent with that policy. Although Heston was an adult, she was temporarily incompetent; competency, not the patient's age, is what is crucial. And as in the other cases, a guardian does not have the right to refuse lifesaving medical treatment for an incompetent.

Things might have been different had Delores Heston previously expressed her wishes while competent. A case like that occurred in Illinois in 1964.[13] Bernice Brooks entered an Illinois hospital in 1964 suffering from a peptic ulcer. She and her husband had informed their family physician, Gilbert Demange, repeatedly over a two-year period that they were Jehovah's Witnesses and that their religious convictions prohibited them from receiving blood transfusions. The Brookses even signed documents releasing Demange and the hospital of all liability that might ensue because blood was not administered. Brooks's condition worsened, and she was no longer able to speak for herself. Her condition was such that if blood were not administered, she would die. Her husband's consent was sought, but, acting on her behalf, he refused to give permission for the administration of blood. Demange petitioned the court, and a legal guardian was appointed who consented to the treatment. Brooks's life was saved. After her recovery, however, she challenged the court order. She won her suit. It was ruled that she had unequivocally expressed her wishes *while competent* and that since her refusal would harm no one else, her right to religious freedom had been violated.

Neither Delores Heston nor Bernice Brooks was competent at the time treatment decisions had to be made, and each was a Jehovah's Witness. The relevant difference between the two cases is that Brooks had expressed her wishes while competent repeatedly and in writing. And, according to the court ruling, such an expression of one's preferences must be honored.

The second type of case is when a guardian refuses treatment for an incompetent that is desirable but not necessary to preserve the patient's life. Again, we shall focus on the case of parents and children. Are parents permitted to refuse treatment for their children that would enhance their children's quality of life but is not necessary to save life? This issue is difficult, both legally and morally. One important question raised here concerns the nature and extent of parental rights. There are limits on what parents may do regarding their children; for example, they may not refuse lifesaving treatment for them in normal circumstances. On the other hand, there are limits on what the state may do in interfering with the lives of children. Certainly states may not force parents to raise their children in any particular religious tradition. But how do we strike a balance here?

Robert Veatch describes a case that brings the difficult issues here to the fore.[14] A fourteen-year-old boy, Jim Powley, was on vacation with his parents and three siblings. As they were driving to a cabin they had rented, they were involved in a serious accident. Powley's father and two older brothers were killed; his mother and sister were badly cut but escaped permanent injury. The boy's leg was severely injured; his femur was broken in two places, and his thigh muscle and hip were crushed. Powley was hospitalized for several months, and his leg began to heal. At this point, his orthopedist recommended corrective surgery. In soliciting Mrs. Powley's permission to perform the surgery, he explained the benefits and risks to her. With the surgery, her son had an excellent chance of regaining the complete use of his leg, though perhaps walking with a slight limp. Without the surgery, there was a 90 percent chance he would lose the use of his leg for life. The greatest risk was from the general anesthesia, which had a risk of one death in several thousand. Mrs. Powley was still recovering from the deaths of her husband and two sons; the mere thought of endangering this boy's life was horrifying to her. Therefore, she refused to give permission to operate, saying instead, "God's will be done." Powley said that he agreed with his mother.

Though not necessary to save Jim Powley's life, this surgery was obviously desirable. With it, Powley had an excellent chance of regaining the use of his leg, which would give him many options that he would otherwise be denied. So we must ask whether it is appropriate to restrict Mrs. Powley's freedom and impose treatment on her son against her wishes, and against his.

The legal status of a guardian's refusal of desirable nonlifesaving treatment is not completely clear. It does appear, however, that what is at work here is a standard of reasonableness.[15] If parents or other legal guardians make a good-faith effort to determine what is best for their child, then their decision will be honored unless it is clearly beyond the bounds of reason. Parents who choose no schooling at all for their children, for example, will have exceeded the bounds of reason. Of course, what is within the bounds of reason is hard to say. However, parental refusal of desirable treatment has been regarded as within the bounds of reason in three types of cases: if the recommended treatment is risky (for example, surgery with a high probability of death), if it is not obvious that the treatment is needed (for example, physicians disagree about the likely efficacy of the treatment), or if treatment can be delayed until the child is of legal age to consent because the treatment administered will still be helpful.[16]

In the case of Jim Powley, none of these three conditions obtains. The treatment proposed is not risky in any ordinary sense of that term. The value and necessity of the treatment are not controversial; Powley will be able to live a much more satisfying life if the surgery is performed successfully. And the treatment cannot be delayed until he becomes an adult; it will be too late then. Even thinking about this case from the moral perspective leaves one with some ambivalence. Considerations that favor intervening include the facts that the proposed treatment is likely to promote Powley's long-term interests and that the mother's expressed wishes are not completely rational due to her depression. But considerations that oppose intervention include the facts that we are reluctant to infringe on parental rights and that such a policy may give health care practitioners and/or the state too much power over familial matters. Here we can say that unless a decision is clearly outside the bounds of reason, parental refusal is normally honored.

Exceptions Regarding Parental Refusal of Life-Sustaining Treatment

As noted earlier, normally a guardian may not refuse lifesaving treatment for an incompetent. The guardian's wishes will be overridden, and the rationale for doing so is the harm principle. But at least two types of cases are exceptions to this rule.

The famous case of Karen Quinlan is an instance of the first type of exception.[17] In April 1975, Quinlan, age twenty-one, lapsed into a persistent vegetative state, apparently as a result of ingesting alcohol and tranquilizers. To sustain her life, she was placed on a respirator. After six months, Joseph Quinlan, her father, petitioned the court to be appointed her guardian for the purpose of discontinuing all extraordinary means of sustaining her life. Physicians at the hospital opposed Quinlan's request. They argued that life-sustaining treatment—in this case, the respirator— should not be discontinued. They predicted that if the woman were taken off the respirator, she would die immediately.

It is interesting to note that the Quinlan case, like that of Delores Heston, occurred in New Jersey. Judge Robert Muir, of the Superior Court of New Jersey, ruled against Quinlan's petition and was apparently influenced by the Heston case. Judge Muir's decision was ultimately reversed by the Supreme Court of New Jersey in January 1976. The Supreme Court of New Jersey gave guardianship to Joseph Quinlan and ruled that the respirator could be turned off at his request. The hospital and the woman's physicians stalled and in the meantime weaned her from the respirator. It was not until May 22, 1976, that she was declared off the respirator, and, contrary to initial predictions, she did not die. Quinlan was then transferred to a public nursing home. She was given artificial nutrition and hydration and antibiotics to protect against infection. Karen Quinlan did not die until June 11, 1985.

The Quinlans were allowed to refuse what doctors said was life-sustaining treatment for their daughter. This is an exception to the usual rule. What is the basis for this? The actual reasoning of the Supreme Court of New Jersey is rather confusing.[18] They appeal to the right to privacy, and it is not clear that such a right is relevant here. Perhaps what is crucial, though, is the court's claim that "no external compelling interest of the State could compel Karen to endure the unendurable, only to vegetate a few measurable months with no realistic possibility of returning to any semblance of cognitive or sapient life." Whether Quinlan's state could be described as "unendurable" is doubtful; all evidence suggests that she experienced no pain. But to say that the state had no compelling interest in forcing her continued treatment can be defended within the framework discussed earlier.

The reason that parents are normally not permitted to refuse lifesaving treatment for incompetents is based on the harm principle; denial of such treatment harms the incompetent. But in some cases, denial of life-extending treatment may not harm the incompetent. In particular, if the patient is in a persistent vegetative state or irreversibly comatose, then arguably death is not a harm for that patient. Viewed in this way, the

Quinlan decision makes sense. The rationale that allows the state to override parental refusal of lifesaving treatment for a child did not exist in the Quinlan case. If a person can never regain consciousness, it is hard to see how death can be regarded as a harm for that person.

A second type of exception to the usual rule concerns treatment for severely defective newborns. These are infants with multiple, life-threatening problems. In some of these cases, parents have been permitted to refuse treatment that might extend the infant's life. Many examples of such multiple afflictions are possible. One scenario concerns severely afflicted myelomeningocele infants.[19] Such infants have an abnormality in the spinal cord that protrudes from the back. They are paralyzed, lack control of the bladder and bowels, and risk a blocked flow of cerebrospinal fluid. As a result, fluid is trapped in the ventricles of the brain, producing swelling and mental retardation. A shunt must be inserted to provide passageway for this fluid. Operations must be performed repeatedly. If they are not performed, the infant will almost certainly die. If the cord abnormality is corrected, some of these babies will live, though with serious physical and mental disabilities and subject to repeated surgeries. In some of these cases, parental refusal of the surgery has been regarded as reasonable.

One way of looking at these cases is this. Unlike the Quinlan case, death for these infants may be regarded as a harm; but death is the lesser of two evils. This is because these infants' continued existence will be painful for them. From the subjects' own perspectives, the burdens of the treatment outweigh the benefits. Judgments of this sort must be made on a case-by-case basis. But when the burdens of treatment do outweigh the benefits, the harm principle does not direct others to compel treatment against the parents' wishes.

One type of case sometimes subsumed under this second exception is controversial. This concerns infants with Down's syndrome, a genetic abnormality in which infants are mentally retarded in varying degrees but not in pain. Sometimes these neonates have other medical problems. And so it was in a case known as "Infant Doe, Indiana," so labeled to preserve the family's anonymity.[20] In April 1982, this infant was born in Bloomington, Indiana, with Down's syndrome and a blocked esophagus. As a result of the blocked esophagus, the infant could not ingest nutrition or hydration. The blocked esophagus could be corrected with surgery, but the parents refused to consent. The hospital's attorney contacted a circuit court judge about this matter, which sustained the parents' decision. The Indiana Supreme Court refused to take the appeal, and the infant died, presumably of dehydration or starvation, before an appeal to the United States Supreme Court could be made.

It is difficult to comment on this case because court records have been sealed, preventing the public from having access to information considered by the court. Two significantly different versions of the case have been told. According to one version, the esophageal problem was easily correctable and would have been performed had it not been for the boy's retardation. According to a second version, the infant had other significant medical problems, some caused by the blocked esophagus, and even with surgery would have suffered greatly. From the moral point of view, it makes all of the difference in the world which of these versions is correct. If the first version is accurate, the parents should not have been allowed to refuse the surgical correction. The infant's retardation is not relevant. Down's syndrome children can and do live contented lives. Parents should be permitted to refuse lifesaving treatment only if the burdens of the treatment and continued existence outweigh the benefits for the patient. If the second version of this case is correct, then perhaps the refusal was warranted. The point that is crucial is whether overall the medical intervention serves the incompetent's interests. The mere existence of an abnormality does not show that the incompetent would not benefit from the treatment; the abnormality has to be such that the incompetent would suffer even after the intervention.

Exceptions Regarding Refusal by a Competent Patient

As explained earlier, a competent patient may refuse any medical treatment, including lifesaving treatment, and for any reason. But are there any exceptions?

One class of exceptions is based on the harm principle. If a person's refusal of treatment will harm other nonconsenting parties, there may be grounds for imposing treatment on that person. We will, of course, have to be careful to explain what constitutes *harm;* the mere fact that another would be saddened by a person's death does not constitute harm to that other. An example that seems uncontroversial here is administering treatment to an unwilling patient with tuberculosis.[21] Here the concern is to prevent the person from exposing others to the disease.

But there are controversial instances of this general exception, all ones involving pregnant patients. In several cases women have been ordered to undergo cesarean sections against their wishes to protect the life of the fetus.[22] The case of Jesse Mae Jefferson occurred in Georgia in 1981. Jefferson was due to deliver her child in several days when the hospital in which she would be attended sought a court order authorizing the performance of a cesarean section and any necessary blood transfusions should she enter the hospital and refuse. Jefferson had placenta previa, and her physician testified that there was a 99 percent chance that her child would not survive vaginal delivery and a 50 percent chance that she herself would not survive it. She had informed the hospital that she had religious objections to cesarean sections and blood transfusions. A Georgia court decided that the unborn child deserved legal protection and authorized the administration of any medical procedures deemed necessary. The court said that the state had a legitimate interest in the preservation of the late-stage fetus's life and that it was a neglected dependent. As it turned out, Jefferson did not go to the hospital and delivered a healthy baby without surgical intervention.

At about the same time, a similar case occurred in Colorado. In this case, the pregnant patient was described as obese, angry, and uncooperative. A fetal heart monitor indicated fetal hypoxia, and a cesarean section was recommended. The patient feared surgery, however, and refused. She was examined and judged competent. The hospital petitioned a juvenile court, the unborn was declared a neglected dependent, and the court ordered the surgery. In this case, the cesarean section was performed, resulting in a healthy baby.

These cases are both exceptional and controversial because the treatment that the patients were required to undergo was highly invasive. It is also regarded as problematic because it interferes with a woman's freedom; normally she chooses her own treatment. No consensus has emerged about the appropriateness of these actions. It is hard to forecast whether there will be more.

A related case that occurred much earlier is worth mentioning here. In 1964 in New Jersey, a pregnant woman refused a blood transfusion necessary to save her life.[23] A court ruled that the unborn fetus is entitled to protection and authorized the performance of the transfusion. This differs somewhat from the cases involving forced cesarean sections because the treatment ordered is less invasive. The underlying principle is the same, however: preventing harm.

A second type of exception to the general rule that competent patients may refuse medical interventions is demonstrated in the well-known case of Elizabeth Bouvia.[24] Bouvia was afflicted with cerebral palsy at birth. Totally dependent on others, she was a quadriplegic and almost totally immobile, except for some very slight movement in one hand and her face. She also suffered from painful arthritis, for which a morphine pump had been implanted in her, and her inability to change her position created muscular pain.

Bouvia had had a very difficult life. Her parents divorced when she was five years old, and her mother placed her in a children's home when she was ten. When she was eighteen, her father told her that he could no longer support her. Bouvia was intelligent and resilient. She had dropped out of high school, but she later completed her general equivalency degree and in 1981 graduated from San Diego State University. She entered a master's program in social work at San Diego State but left in 1982 over a disagreement about her fieldwork placement.

Bouvia's difficulties continued. In August 1982, she married Richard Bouvia shortly after he was released from prison. They had been corresponding by mail. They conceived a child, but Bouvia suffered a miscarriage. Her husband had difficulties getting a job, and efforts to secure financial assistance from various family members failed. In 1983 the Bouvias were living in Oregon, where Bouvia's parents resided, when her husband abandoned her. At this point, she asked her father to drive her to California, where she was still a legal resident.

In September 1983, Bouvia admitted herself to the psychiatric ward of Riverside (California) General Hospital. As a resident, she was eligible for Medi-Cal. Unbeknownst to the staff there, she planned to commit suicide by starving herself to death. She informed the staff that she would not eat and asked that they give her pain medication and maintain her hygiene. The hospital indicated that they would not assist her in committing suicide and that if she continued to refuse food, they would force-feed her through a nasogastric tube. Bouvia sought a court order to prevent this procedure. She argued that her rights of privacy and self-determination prohibited the hospital from initiating such invasive procedures. Donald Fisher, Riverside's chief of psychiatry, opposed going along with Bouvia's wishes, saying, "Sometimes to focus on somebody's rights is to get in the way of their [sic] well-being."

The court ruled in favor of the hospital, refusing to grant Bouvia's request. The issue of her competence had been raised by the hospital, but, based on the testimony of consulting psychiatrists, Judge John Hews said that she was sincere, rational, and fully competent. During this time, many people with disabilities held vigils designed to get Bouvia to change her mind. They feared that her actions would promote the view that all people with disabilities are better off dead. In siding with the hospital, Judge Hews was concerned about the "profound effect on the medical staff, nurses, and administration of the hospital" and the "devastating effect on other . . . physically handicapped persons" if Bouvia were allowed to starve herself to death.[25]

The relevance of the effects on other people with disabilities is highly doubtful. But there is a way to explain the rationale underlying this decision without denying that competent patients have a right to refuse any medical treatment.[26] What Elizabeth Bouvia was denied in this case was the right to demand and receive assistance from others in ending her life.

Health care practitioners cannot be forced to assist a person in committing suicide. Bouvia's right to self-determination gave her a right to check out of the hospital but not a right to require health care professionals to participate in her plan on hospital turf. Competent patients do not have a right to demand anything they want, and health care workers have a right to withdraw from cases to which they have moral objections. If the relationship between competent patients and health care providers is conceived in terms of the contractual model, neither party may be forced to act against her own principles. Had Bouvia been forthright about her intentions, it is unlikely that health care providers would have agreed to her terms. So understood, this case does not deviate from the usual rulings regarding competent patients.[27]

There is a third type of exception regarding competent patients who will not consent to treatment. Judges have sometimes allowed physicians to treat patients who will not explicitly consent but who let it be known that they will not actively resist. This was the situation in 1965 in the case of Willie Mae Powell in New York. Powell had refused to consent to a blood transfusion but apparently made it known that she would not put up resistance if blood were administered to her. She had signed a release of liability. Her husband petitioned for a court order for the transfusion. In issuing the order, Judge Jacob Markowitz said, "This woman wanted to live. I could not let her die!"[28] Such a decision appears to invoke paternalism. In particular, the judge claims to know what the patient really wants in spite of the patient's refusal to confirm this opinion.

A fourth type of exception, related to the first, will be mentioned briefly; it is illustrated in a case involving Jesse E. Jones.[29] Jones, age twenty-five with a seven-month-old child, was brought to the hospital for emergency care by her husband. She had lost significant amounts of blood due to a ruptured ulcer. With her life in jeopardy, the hospital sought permission to administer blood. Her husband refused to consent. Judge J. Skelly Wright quickly arranged a bedside hearing. All that he could understand Jones saying was, "Against my will." Nevertheless, he ordered the transfusion. Among the reasons he gave to justify this decision were appeals to the interests of the child and the mother's obligations to it. This is like the first exception in that the interests of others override the patient's refusal. But in cases of the first sort, the child's life was at stake. Here any harm that will come to the child due to the parent's refusal of treatment is more speculative and remote.

So, though a competent patient has a right to refuse medical therapy, including lifesaving treatment, there are some exceptions.[30] These exceptions are rare.

THE ELEMENTS OF INFORMED CONSENT

In addition to the right to refuse treatment, normally no medical intervention may be initiated without the competent patient's consent. Though this is a complicated topic,[31] here we shall try to explain the main elements of informed consent.[32]

Competence is a presupposition of obtaining informed consent. Only competent patients can autonomously authorize treatment. The fundamental meaning of "competence" is the ability to perform a task. We use the terms *competence* and *incompetence* as if they were global, all-or-nothing terms. But clearly competence varies from context to context; one may be competent to perform some tasks but not others. In medical contexts what must be decided is whether patients are competent to make their own medical decisions. Even this issue may be context-dependent. For some hold that as a medical intervention increases the risks for persons, the level of ability required for a judgment of competence to accept or refuse the intervention should also be increased. Judgments about competence are often difficult.

The second element of informed consent is *disclosure of information*. This item is what the courts have focused on, and we shall discuss it further later. Here we shall note that the information that health care practitioners must provide patients to ensure informed consent include at least the following: the potential or likely risks associated with the treatment; the alternatives, if any, to the recommended treatment and the risks associated with them; and the likely results if the patient chooses to forgo treatment.

Understanding is the third element of informed consent. The idea here is to try to make sure that the patient has grasped the information that has been presented. It is one thing to present information and quite another for those to whom it is presented to grasp it. Morally responsible health care professionals must be aware of factors that can impair or hinder understanding. These factors include irrationality, immaturity, and information overload. Sometimes patients simply need time to absorb the information presented, although that is not always a luxury available in medical contexts. And sometimes how information is presented can make a difference. When there is time to determine understanding, some experienced health care professionals report a useful technique. Instead of asking patients *whether* they understand what they have been told, these physicians and nurses ask the patients to tell them *what* they understand about their condition and the treatments being offered. Patients are sometimes reticent to acknowledge their ignorance; this technique can provide a graceful way of determining the need for more explanation.

The fourth element of informed consent is *voluntariness*. The idea here is to make sure that the patient has not been pressured into agreeing to treatment. Acceptance or rejection of treatment must be the competent patient's own decision. One obstacle to the voluntariness of consent is coercion, such as applying pressure or threatening the patient. Another obstacle to voluntariness is manipulation, which can occur if patients are given only selected information so that they will agree to the recommended treatment.

The final element of informed consent is *authorization*. This means that the patient has said yes and/or has signed the requisite forms signifying approval.

While these five elements can be distinguished in theory, in practice things can get quite messy. A case involving a sixty-year-old Greek immigrant illustrates some of the difficulties. This woman was hospitalized with a gangrenous foot but refused the recommended amputation. Late one afternoon, Dr. R's intern paged him and told him that he must examine this woman. Her foot was black and cold, her leg was red and hot, and she was terrified. The intern informed Dr. R that the patient would not consent to the operation. As Dr. R spoke to the patient, she begged him repeatedly to wash her foot. Antibiotics and morphine gave the patient relief from pain and septicemia, but without the amputation she would die within a few weeks.

By an incredible coincidence, Dr. R's intern that night was a second-generation Greek American well-versed in the culture, religion, and language of his ancestry. He conversed with the patient in Greek. There was no doubt that in many ways she was mentally competent. She was a virtual recluse with no family and spoke very poor English. Her former employer, an elderly Greek man, was called in to talk with her, but neither he nor the intern could reason with her about the danger she was in. Dr. R and the intern went so far as to demonstrate to her that the blackness could not be removed with soap and water, but still she remained adamant against amputation. The intern pointed out that this woman was originally from a rural village where all major decisions were made by one's father or a village elder. He suspected that this woman was emotionally paralyzed by her cultural isolation.[33]

A certainty was evident about this case seldom present in medicine: without the amputation this woman would die, and with it she would live. Dr. R would have honored this woman's wishes had she said, "I understand what you are saying, but I do not want to live with one leg." But nothing like that was communicated by her. Dr. R sought and received a court order, and he amputated her leg. The next morning the patient was smiling and profoundly relieved. What is interesting about this case is that the woman was in most respects competent. The problem here seemed to be her inability to understand the situation and perhaps her reluctance to make major decisions. Cultural factors adversely affected her understanding. That condition certainly did not make her globally incompetent, but perhaps it made her incompetent to make major medical decisions. What seems to be true here is that the elements of competence and understanding are intertwined in ways that are difficult to sort out.

THE COURTS AND INFORMED CONSENT

In dealing with informed consent, the courts have tended to focus on two items: disclosure of information and authorization. Two cases in 1972 have been influential in shaping legal discussions of informed consent: *Canterbury v. Spence* (Washington, D.C.) and *Cobbs v. Grant* (California).[34]

In *Canterbury v. Spence*, John Canterbury, a nineteen-year-old, developed paraplegia after a laminectomy. Before surgery, his physician, William Spence, did not inform Canterbury that the operation involved a risk of paralysis. Spence said that he did not tell the patient about the 1 percent chance of paralysis because "it is not good medical practice"—it might deter patients from undergoing needed surgery. Canterbury sued. Judge Spottswood Robinson ruled that "every human being of adult years and sound mind has a right to determine what shall be done to his own body" and that therefore patients must be adequately informed so that they can evaluate their options knowledgeably. This ruling requires physicians to warn patients about the risks of the recommended treatment, the available alternatives, if any, and the likely consequences of refusing treatment.

In *Cobbs v. Grant*, Ralph Cobbs was admitted to the hospital for treatment of a duodenal ulcer. He was given medication for discomfort but still complained. Surgery was recommended. The surgeon, Dudley Grant, explained the nature of the operation with Cobbs but did not discuss any of the inherent risks. Nine days after the apparently successful surgery, Cobbs began to experience abdominal pain. Internal bleeding was discovered, the result of an artery near the spleen that was accidentally severed during the previous surgery. Additional surgery was needed. A month later, Cobbs again experienced sharp pains in his stomach. He was developing another ulcer. Again, surgery was needed. Neither the possibility of a severed artery nor the possibility of the recurrence of an ulcer was explained to the patient; yet each of these is a risk associated with the original surgery. The California Supreme Court, using language similar to that of Judge Robinson, affirmed that physicians have a duty to inform patients of possible risks associated with any recommended treatment. And like Judge Robinson, they cited the patient's right to self-determination as the basis for such a duty.

It should be pointed out that in both *Canterbury v. Spence* and *Cobbs v. Grant*, the courts demanded that the patients prove that failure to disclose a risk was the "cause" of the injury. To establish this point, the patients had to show that disclosure of the relevant material risk would have resulted in a decision against treatment. Of course, patients' own testimony to this effect is likely to be unconvincing, since they have the advantage of hindsight and self-interested reasons to say that they would have decided differently. So what must be shown is that a "prudent person" in the patient's position would have decided differently if adequately informed.[35]

But what risks must a physician explain to a patient? It would be practically impossible to explain *every possible* risk. But then on what basis do physicians determine what risks to disclose? The courts in both *Canterbury v. Spence* and *Cobbs v. Grant* address this very difficult issue. Previously the criterion employed to determine what physicians should tell their patients was medical custom, meaning that any individual physician should do what most other physicians in similar situations do. But the courts in these two cases explicitly reject medical custom as the proper test for determining what risks to disclose. One reason to reject this criterion is that it can lead to the perpetuation of pervasive negligence; that is, if most physicians were engaged in a practice that adversely affected patients, this criterion would permit its continuation.

In addition, this criterion ignores the rights of patients. But what is recommended in its place? The courts in these two cases endorse what has come to be known as "the reasonable person standard." This guideline tells physicians that they must disclose a possible risk if the "average reasonable person" in the patient's position would want to have that information in making a decision. This standard, while regarded by most as superior to medical custom, still has problems. It is difficult to apply the standard in many cases. In some cases, it is far from obvious what information the mythical reasonable person would deem essential to making an informed decision. As a result, this standard does not give health care practitioners precise guidance in these difficult cases.

Some have urged the adoption of a more subjective standard. According to this view, health care professionals should disclose the information that the particular patient would regard as relevant. This recommendation is problematic, however, because it requires health care providers to have more knowledge of the idiosyncracies of their patients than is reasonable to expect. Frequently today, patients are treated by specialists with whom they have had little or no previous interaction. In these situations, one can hardly expect the health care professionals to know what information their particular patients would deem important. So even with the rejection of medical custom as the standard for determining what information to give to patients, difficulties remain, for problems persist with both the reasonable person standard and the subjective criterion.

The five elements that are components of informed consent in the moral sense make most sense within the framework of the contractual model of the health care practitioner–patient relationship. We should emphasize that within this model, patients who want to be fully informed have obligations and must play an active role in the process. For example, sometimes they must ask questions. But, as noted in the previous chapter, some patients do not want to play a role in their own medical decisions. These patients are sometimes said to have *waived* their right to informed consent; they have given physicians permission to treat them without securing informed consent. Waiver is regarded by many as one of the legitimate exceptions to the requirement of informed consent.[36]

There is, however, a more controversial exception to the doctrine of informed consent, an exception endorsed in *Canterbury v. Spence* and *Cobbs v. Grant*. This exception is referred to as *the therapeutic privilege*. As Judge Robinson puts it, it allows physicians to withhold information "when risk disclosure poses such a threat of detriment to the patient as to become unfeasible or contraindicated from a medical point of view." This exception allows physicians to withhold information about risks for paternalistic reasons.

Obviously, allowing such an exception conflicts with the emphasis on self-determination that is the very ground on which the doctrine of informed consent rests. Some doubt that the therapeutic privilege should be extended to physicians when patients are competent. Judge Robinson himself recognizes the problem. He says that the "physician's privilege to withhold information for therapeutic reasons must be carefully circumscribed, however, for otherwise it might devour the disclosure rule itself." But exactly how it is to be circumscribed is not clear. As a result, some worry that merely allowing the therapeutic privilege puts us on a slippery slope that ends in the very paternalism that the doctrine of informed consent was designed to oppose. This remains a controversy.

TREATMENT WITHOUT CONSENT: THE MORAL ISSUE

As we have seen, it is legally permissible to administer emergency treatment to an incompetent patient when no one is available to speak for the patient. The moral principle underlying this is weak paternalism. And it is legally permissible to override a guardian's refusal of lifesaving treatment for an incompetent; the harm principle is the basis for such intervention. It is also permissible to treat competent patients against their wishes when doing so is necessary to prevent harm to other innocent parties. Examples include forcing immunization against a contagious disease or quarantining persons. But is it ever morally permissible to treat competent patients without their consent for their own good? If it is, the underlying principle would seem to be strong paternalism. Here we shall investigate this possibility.

Let us begin by distinguishing three different kinds of cases of treating competent patients without consent for their own good. Some consensus exists about how the first two types of cases should be handled, but the third holds some uncertainty. The approach here will be to compare the first two cases with the third for the purpose of seeing how the third should be handled. This study will provide a basis for more general conclusions about the issue of treatment without consent.

The first kind of case—hereafter called cases of type 1—involves patients who have neither consented nor refused treatment. Some evidence indicates that both the medical and legal communities approve of treatment without consent in at least some cases of this sort. As noted earlier, the courts have dealt with some of these cases. Recall the example of Willie Mae Powell. For religious reasons, she would not consent to a needed blood transfusion. But she made it known that she would not actively resist, either. The judge allowed the administration of blood in this case. Recall, too, that in *Canterbury v. Spence*, Judge Robinson allowed for cases in which the therapeutic privilege might be invoked. This privilege allows physicians to administer treatment without fully informed consent if in their judgment soliciting consent is medically inadvisable. The medical community has also approved of such intervention, specifically in some of its official pronouncements about therapeutic experiments. A therapeutic experiment is one in which a new or untested drug or medical procedure is employed and the primary goal is to help the patient in question; typically, all standard therapy in such cases has failed or is contraindicated. In some circumstances, a physician may judge that if information about the experimental procedure or drug is revealed to the patient, that patient's health will be adversely affected; that is, disclosure is contrary to the patient's best interests. Approval of treatment without consent in this type of situation is suggested in Part II of the "Declaration of Helsinki" (first drafted in 1964 and revised in 1975) and is stated explicitly in the "American Medical Association Ethical Guidelines for Clinical Investigations" (originally adopted in 1966).[37] There is, then, some consensus about cases of type 1.

The second kind of case—hereafter type 2—arises when a patient explicitly objects to a specific kind of treatment. The objection is usually for religious reasons, though it need not be. The familiar case of the Jehovah's Witness who refuses a blood transfusion is an example. But if a competent patient with a gangrenous foot refuses the recommended amputation because she does not want to live without all limbs, normally that refusal must be honored; religion plays no role here. As we have seen, the law in the United States says that competent patients have a right to refuse any medical treatment, and physicians who fail to respect this right may be guilty of battery. And though initially resistant, now members of the medical community seem to accept the principle of autonomy and the fact that it gives competent patients the right to refuse recommended medical interventions, even when that refusal seems foolish. A recent nursing journal reports a case, for instance, in which a young man becomes a quadriplegic as the result of a diving accident.[38] After a few months of ups and downs, he decides to refuse all medical treatment. He is sent home and dies. Commentators on this case see his decision as unfortunate but agree that his wishes needed to be respected.

There is a third kind of case—type 3—in which the issue of treatment without consent arises. This situation arises when a patient refuses a specific form of treatment because of a false belief. The patient's refusal is based on neither religion nor an aversion to the particular treatment; rather, the patient is mistaken about certain factual aspects of the case. An interesting example of this sort involves a woman who was hospitalized because of a fractured hip.[39] A Papanicolaou test that analyzes cells from the cervix and vagina for cancer and a biopsy revealed that this woman had cervical cancer. Physicians judged that the cancer was curable by a hysterectomy and so recommended this surgery. The patient refused to consent to this procedure, however; in spite of the evidence, she did not believe that she had cancer. She said that people with cancer feel bad and lose weight, and these conditions did not hold in her case.

Assuming that the patient is judged competent, we are presented with a difficult problem: Is paternalistic intervention justified in this case? Most will agree that in cases of this sort, physicians have an obligation to try to change the patients' beliefs so that they can make an informed decision. But if that fails, may a specific kind of treatment be forced on patients if their only reason for refusing is that they have false beliefs about the facts?

Initially cases of type 3 are the troublesome ones; there is some consensus about types 1 and 2. To get a handle on type 3 cases, let us compare them with types 1 and 2 and see which they resemble more. The ultimate goal here is to uncover and examine critically a rationale supporting paternalism in cases of type 3. We will go through three stages of comparison, the third of which will include criticisms of the paternalistic rationale.

For the first stage of this comparative inquiry, consider the most glaring difference between type 1 and type 2 cases. In cases of type 1, the patient has simply *not consented* to the treatment; but in cases of type 2 the patient has *explicitly refused* the recommended treatment. If health care practitioners were to impose treatment in each of these cases, the magnitude of the interference would differ in the two. It is a more serious invasion of autonomy to go against the explicit wishes of a person than it is merely to do something to a person without that person's consent. Interference in type 2 cases is more serious than that in type 1 cases. This is an important difference. In this respect, cases of type 3 are more like those of type 2 than type 1; for the patient has also explicitly refused treatment in type 3 cases. So a superficial comparison of the cases suggests that cases of type 3 should be handled like those of type 2, which requires that refusal be respected.

But such an analysis seems too superficial and invites us to take the comparative inquiry to a second stage. For interfering with the Jehovah's Witness who has refused a blood transfusion seems much more difficult to justify than interfering with the woman who does not believe that she has cervical cancer, even though most think that both have false beliefs. Not only that, in some cases paternalistic action regarding one who has a false belief seems permissible. Note the case of Mill's man, mentioned earlier, who is prepared to cross the dangerous bridge. Even Mill, an opponent of paternalism, thinks that detaining the man is warranted. These observations suggest that there are morally relevant differences between type 2 and type 3 cases, and so a deeper examination of the cases is in order.

What really bothers us about treatment without consent in cases of type 2? Why is there such a consensus about these cases? If we were to engage in treatment without consent in cases of type 2, we would be *imposing our values* on the patient. We would be saying that the patient's values either do not count or are overridden by ours. And we are properly quite reluctant to impose our values on others; we avoid this if morally possible. But if we engage in treatment without consent in type 1 cases, would we be imposing our values on the patient? This question can be answered in the negative.

Health care practitioners who invoke the therapeutic privilege and judges who approve of this seem to analyze type 1 cases in the following way. The patient has come to the health care professional for help and wants what is medically best. The end is to do what is medically best for the patient, and the only question concerns the means to that end. If the physician judges that the end can only be achieved by initiating treatment without fully informed consent, then such action is permissible. So understood, physicians are *not* imposing their values on patients when they engage in treatment without consent in cases of type 1. On the contrary, they are *helping patients get what they really want*. For the patient wants to get better, and the only question is about the means.

Continuing this comparative inquiry at this second stage, are cases of type 3 more like those of type 2 or type 1? If treatment without consent is initiated in type 3 cases, would health care professionals be imposing their values on the patients? This question can be answered in the negative, and so in spite of initial appearances, cases of type 3 are more like those of type 1 than type 2. If the woman with cervical cancer really values her life and health, then she wants to preserve them.[40] And if so, then if she correctly believed that she had the illness, she would consent to the surgery needed to arrest it. So if health care workers interfere and force treatment on her, they will be forcing her to do what she would *really want* if her factual beliefs about the case were correct. So in some sense they would be forcing her to do what she really wants. And in the most difficult cases of type 1, where the Jehovah's Witness will not consent but will not actively oppose treatment, judges have said, perhaps mistakenly, that treatment is what the patient really wants. In the case of Willie Mae Powell, Judge Markowitz said, "This woman wanted to live. I could not let her die."[41]

Notice that this same analysis applies to Mill's man. He was about to cross a bridge, not knowing that doing so was dangerous. He did not want to fall into the river and be hurt. In fact, in discussing this case, Mill appeals to the same rationale we have been discussing. He suggests that stopping the man from crossing the bridge is not really interfering with his liberty. This point depends on a particular analysis of liberty, one provided by Mill: "Liberty consists in doing what one desires." Some clarification is needed here, however, because the expression "doing what one desires" is ambiguous. On the one hand, "doing what one desires" may refer to the description under which an object is desired. This is called the *intended* object of desire. On the other hand, "what one desires" may refer to the real object of a desire, whether or not one knows that it is the object of desire. This is called the *actual* object of desire.[42]

The intended and actual objects of desire will be different whenever the agent has false beliefs about what is desired. Thus, if a person mistakes a plastic, imitation apple for a real apple and desires to eat it, the *intended* object of desire is to eat a real apple, and the *actual* object of desire is to eat the plastic apple. Though Mill's analysis of liberty is subject to this ambiguity, what he goes on to say—"he does not desire to fall into the river"—clarifies what he means. "Liberty consists in doing what one desires" means that liberty consists of doing or acquiring the *intended* object of a desire. Thus, in cases of a false belief, when a person is prevented from seeking the actual object of a desire, that person's liberty is not really interfered with.

So there is a common rationale to justify treatment without consent in cases of type 1 and 3; in each case, one claims that treatment is what the patient really wants. So treatment in these two cases does not wrongly interfere; it actually promotes the patient's own values and liberty, when liberty is understood in Mill's way.

The third and final stage of this comparative inquiry is to ask whether the rationale just explained to justify treatment without consent in cases of types 1 and 3 is plausible. One can argue that the consequences of accepting this rationale are undesirable, and the account of liberty on which it is based is implausible. Three points are paramount. First, allowing others to force a person to do something because they believe it will lead to what the person really wants does not ensure that the intended object of desire will be achieved. Others, including health care providers, can never be sure what another person's real wishes are. Still, a defender of the rationale might object that in the cases in question, there can be no doubt about what the person really wants; the person has a false belief about the means necessary to achieve the desirable end.

We can easily exaggerate our knowledge of what another wants. But even granting the response to the first objection, a second point against accepting the rationale emerges. Permitting intervention on the basis of this rationale will open the door to far too much paternalism; indeed, it practically gives health care practitioners a blank check. On this basis, one can argue for the involuntary sterilization of mentally retarded teenagers. After all, the argument goes, what they really want from life is happiness, and whether they realize it or not, they cannot be happy if they are saddled with children who themselves may be retarded. Even more surprising, this rationale can be employed to force Jehovah's Witnesses to receive blood transfusions. The end that Jehovah's Witnesses seek is to obey God's law, but, it will be argued, they mistakenly believe that God's law requires the refusal of blood transfusions. Interference will enable them to attain the intended object of their desire. In general, then, it appears that many type 2 cases can be subsumed under the rationale used to justify treatment without consent in type 1 and 3 cases. This point is a reason to reject the rationale.

We should be wary of this rationale for a third reason—namely, because it erroneously assumes that people only care about the ends they achieve. But this view is a mistake; people also care about how those ends are achieved. You may want a certain job very much, for example, but you do not want to get it because of your race, gender, or relationship with the boss. You want to get it because you are the best qualified; to get it for any other reason is an affront to your dignity. Some might grant this point in the abstract but contend that it has no applicability in medical contexts. After all, people want good health and are not concerned about how they achieve that end. But that argument is a mistake. Certainly Jehovah's Witnesses do not want to achieve good health if that requires the administration of blood. And many may want to have a say in how the end is achieved.

These criticisms suggest that the most obvious rationale to justify treatment without consent in cases of type 3 is inadequate. But consider again Mill's man. He has a false belief, and most of us approve of paternalistic intervention in that case. So why should we not interfere in the medical cases, too? The answer to this question is that there are important differences between Mill's case and the typical type 3 case in medicine. Two differences will be highlighted here.

First, immediate physical intervention is necessary with Mill's man because there is no time to reason with him or warn him. The purpose of the intervention is to buy such time; the harm cannot be prevented without the intervention. But in many medical cases, there is time to reason with the patient. In the case of the woman with cervical cancer, health care providers and family members were able to persuade her of the reality of the cancer, and she then consented to the needed treatment.

Second, interference with Mill's man is only temporary. Once the dangers have been pointed out to him, then he is free to cross if he wishes and further interference is not warranted, assuming that he is competent. But in many medical cases, if patients are treated without consent, the interference is irrevocable. Health care practitioners cannot remove transfused blood, or replace an amputated limb, or undo a hysterectomy. In short, those detaining Mill's man are engaged in weak paternalism. But imposing treatment without consent in many of the type 3 cases will be strongly paternalistic.

The law gives competent patients a right to refuse medical treatment, and its basis is in a person's right to self-determination. The argument here gives three reasons for rejecting a common rationale to support treatment without consent in cases of type 1 and 3. Together, these considerations make a strong case against treatment without consent in all three types of cases (unless there is some other rationale). These considerations urge the rejection of strong paternalism.

But as with our discussion of confidentiality and truth telling, we should ask whether we can really accept an absolute prohibition against strong paternalism. Several cases will be discussed to bring out some of the complexities here.

First, consider the well-known case of Donald C.[43] At age twenty-six, Donald had graduated from college and completed service in the military. At that time he joined his father's real estate business. On July 25, 1973, Donald and his father were appraising farm land. They had unknowingly parked their car near a large propane gas line. When they started the car, the ignition set off an explosion, and the surrounding countryside was engulfed in fire. Donald's father died on the way to the hospital. Donald was admitted to the hospital in a critical but conscious state. He had second- and third-degree burns over 68 percent of his body. Both eyes were blinded by corneal damage, his ears were mostly destroyed, and his face and upper body were severely burned. During the next nine months, Donald underwent repeated skin grafting, amputations of parts of his fingers, and numerous surgeries on his eyes. In April 1974, he was admitted to the University of Texas Medical Branch Hospitals. Because he had many infected areas on his body, he had to bathe daily in the Hubbard tank.

From the day of the accident, Donald said that he did not want to live. He continued to accept treatment, however. But after admission to the university hospital, Donald had reached his limit. He refused to give permission for any more corrective surgery, and he demanded that he be allowed to leave the hospital and return home. If this were to occur, he would die due to the infections. His mother did not want this. The tankings were continued in spite of his protests.

At this point, Robert White, a psychiatric consultant, was asked to see Donald. White was given the impression that Donald was irrational and depressed and probably needed to be declared incompetent so that treatments could be continued. White's assessment, however, was quite different. He said that Donald was smart, articulate, and coherent; he certainly was not incompetent. Donald had simply decided that he did not want to live as a blind and crippled person with severe limitations. And White admitted that if he were in Donald's position, he would probably want to die, too. Yet White was quite concerned about the impact of this decision on Donald's mother, especially if Donald were to die in her home.

White judged that Donald's complete dependence on others was exacerbating the situation. So he offered to help Donald get legal assistance. White said that he and the other physicians at the hospital could not accede to his wishes to leave the hospital because that would be assisting him in suicide and would place an unfair burden on his mother. But,

White said, if the court said that Donald had the right to refuse further treatment, then the hospital would abide by that ruling. And not only that, they agreed that Donald could remain in the hospital until his death. Donald won in court, but then agreed to continue treatment. He made progress and was eventually able to leave the hospital. White believes that gaining some control over his life was what Donald really needed.

By not honoring Donald's refusal of treatment until a court order was given, White and the hospital were treating a competent patient paternalistically (while also trying to protect his mother). But perhaps this was not a case of strong paternalism. Looked at one way, White and the hospital were buying time. They hoped that by giving Donald some control over his situation and more time to reflect, he would change his mind. Delaying a decision in the hope that a patient will reconsider is arguably only weakly paternalistic, at least if the delay is not extensive. And they were prepared to honor Donald's wishes if he did not change his mind. The mere occurrence of a good outcome does not prove that the case was handled properly; even with the good outcome, it may have been inappropriate paternalism. But one suspects that delaying tactics, if not extended too far, are appropriate to ensure that the patient really wants to end the treatment. If that is what went on here, then it is not strong paternalism. Whether the health care practitioners in this case went too far is an important question.

Let us now consider a second case that may challenge the antipaternalistic conclusions reached earlier. Generically, the kind of case one wants here is one in which the well-being of a competent patient can be protected with a minimal invasion of autonomy. Such a case might obtain if one could run an extra diagnostic test without the patient's knowledge. The purpose of running the test is to determine whether the patient has a certain disease. The reason for not informing the patient is that the probability that the patient has the disease is very small, and knowledge that this is even a possibility is likely to upset the patient greatly. Now consider a particular case that falls under this genus.

Mrs. Z is an eighty-year-old widow. She has several medical problems and is receiving regular care from her physician. Three years ago, blood was administered to Mrs. Z during surgery. The blood was obtained from the Red Cross. Mr. Y was the donor. Of course, Mr. Y's blood had been tested and was not contaminated with HIV. The Red Cross just learned, however, that Mr. Y has contracted HIV. The problem is this: Blood can be contaminated, but tests will not reveal this state because the body needs a certain amount of time to develop the antibodies that will be detected by the test. And the amount of time for the body to develop the antibodies varies from person to person. Given the three-year time lapse, it is very unlikely that Mrs. Z received contaminated blood; still, it is possible that she did.

Now suppose that Mrs. Z's physician routinely draws blood from her during her quarterly visits, testing it for various things. The Red Cross has informed the physician about the potential problem. The physician believes that Mrs. Z should be tested for HIV, but he does not want to upset her, especially given how unlikely it is that she is afflicted. He will have a blood sample anyway, and he knows a lab technician who will run the test regardless of legalities. If the test is positive, of course the physician will inform the patient. If the test is negative, he will say nothing. One benefit to the patient is not to alarm her needlessly when the likelihood that she has contracted HIV is so small. The physician thinks that merely informing her of this possibility is likely to cause her great distress. Another benefit is that if she has indeed contracted HIV, she can choose among various therapeutic options. Even though now HIV is incurable, some treatments seem to extend an inflicted patient's life.

If the physician carries out this contemplated option, he will have acted in a strongly paternalistic manner—acting in what he believes is the best interests of a competent patient without her consent. His proposed action is minimally invasive; he will draw blood anyway, and if the test is negative, as expected, nobody will have additional information about Mrs. Z.

Is this option morally acceptable? We shall not try to resolve this issue here but simply note that this case arouses some people's ire because of the emotional baggage surrounding HIV and AIDS. You might do well to change the example slightly and see whether you still have the same reaction. Suppose that instead of testing for HIV, the possible but unlikely medical problem is a form of cancer detectable through a blood test. Everything else about the case is the same. The benefits are not upsetting the patient about something that is very unlikely and giving the patient therapeutic options if the test is positive. In that situation, would doing the additional test without consent be permissible?

SUMMARY

With few exceptions, competent patients have the legal right to refuse medical treatment, even lifesaving treatment. This view affirms the right to self-determination and, at least in this context, rejects strong paternalism. In emergency situations when the patient is not competent and no one is authorized to speak for the patient, health care practitioners have a right to administer any needed medical treatment. This situation affirms the importance of beneficence and is an instance of weak paternalism. If a legal guardian refuses lifesaving treatment for an incompetent patient, normally that refusal is not honored and treatment is administered. Such rulings suggest that, at least in medical contexts, guardians do not have a right to make decisions blatantly contrary to the interests of the dependent.

There are legal exceptions to this rule, however. If the proposed life-sustaining treatment will merely keep the body functioning but offer no benefits because, for example, the patient is in a persistent vegetative state, or the burdens of the treatment outweigh the benefits because of the patient's extreme discomfort, then the guardian's refusal may be honored. When a guardian refuses desirable treatment that is not lifesaving, matters are more difficult. The law seems to handle such situations on a case-by-case basis and tries to determine whether the guardian's refusal is within the bounds of reason when both the benefits and burdens are weighed.

Informed consent can come only from competent patients or the guardians of incompetent patients. For consent to be fully informed, the following elements must be present: (1) the physician must disclose all relevant information to the patient, including the risks associated with the recommended treatment, alternatives to that treatment, and the likely consequences if treatment is refused; (2) the physician must attempt to make sure that the patient has understood the information; (3) the consent must be voluntary and secured without pressure or duress; and (4) the patient must have properly authorized the treatment.

If it is always *morally* wrong to treat a competent patient without fully informed consent, then we reject strong paternalism in medicine. But some situations may give us cause for pause. When a competent patient refuses needed medical treatment because of a false belief, we are tempted to impose treatment. If the patient's refusal is due to some serious misunderstanding, then it is not informed refusal. But a false belief need not always signal a lack of understanding. In that case, imposing treatment without consent is tempting on grounds that this care actually enables patients to get what they really want. However, several criticisms of this rationale were given.

Nevertheless, it is difficult to conclude that treating a competent patient without fully informed consent is always wrong. For situations may arise where the invasiveness is minimal and the potential benefits are great, and in such cases it is not obvious that autonomy always trumps beneficence.

Suggestions for Further Reading

Annas, George J. "Forced Cesareans: The Most Unkindest Cut of All." *The Hastings Center Report*, Vol. 12 (June 1982), pp. 16–17, 45.

Annas, George J. *The Rights of Patients* (Totowa, NJ: Humana, 1992), Chapters 6 and 8.

Beauchamp, Tom L., and James F. Childress. *Principles of Biomedical Ethics*, 4th ed. (New York: Oxford University Press, 1994), pp. 144–170 and 277–291.

Buchanan, Allan E., and Dan W. Brock. *Deciding for Others* (New York: Cambridge University Press, 1989).

Faden, Ruth R., and Alan I. Faden. "False Belief and the Refusal of Medical Treatment." *Journal of Medical Ethics*, Vol. 3 (1977), pp. 133–136.

Faden, Ruth R., and Tom L. Beauchamp. *A History and Theory of Informed Consent* (New York: Oxford University Press, 1986).

Feinberg, Joel. *Harm to Others* (New York: Oxford University Press, 1984).

Feinberg, Joel. "Legal Paternalism." In *Rights, Justice, and the Bounds of Liberty* (Princeton, NJ: Princeton University Press, 1980), pp. 110–129.

Mill, John Stuart. *On Liberty* (Indianapolis: Hackett, 1978). (Originally published in 1859.)

Pence, Gregory E. *Classic Cases in Medical Ethics* (New York: McGraw-Hill, 1990), Chapters 1 and 2.

Underwood, Robert C. "From *In re* Brooks Estate." In Samuel Gorovitz, Ruth Macklin, Andrew Jameton, John O'Connor, and Susan Sherwin (eds.), *Moral Problems in Medicine*, 2d ed. (Upper Saddle River, NJ: Prentice Hall, 1983), pp. 62–63.

Veatch, Robert M. *Case Studies in Medical Ethics* (Cambridge, MA: Harvard University Press, 1977), pp. 303–316.

Veatch, Robert M. *Death, Dying, and the Biological Revolution*, rev. ed. (New Haven, CT: Yale University Press, 1989), Chapters 4 and 5.

Notes

1. The classic presentation of this topic is found in John Stuart Mill, *On Liberty* (Indianapolis: Hackett, 1978).

2. For a thorough study of the harm principle, see Joel Feinberg, *Harm to Others* (New York: Oxford University Press, 1984).

3. See Joel Feinberg, "Legal Paternalism," in *Rights, Justice, and the Bounds of Liberty* (Princeton, NJ: Princeton University Press, 1980), pp. 110–129, and Tom L. Beauchamp and James F. Childress, *Principles of Biomedical Ethics*, 4th ed. (New York: Oxford University Press, 1994), pp. 277–291.

4. Mill, *On Liberty*, Chapter 5.

5. Quoted in Robert M. Veatch, *Death, Dying, and the Biological Revolution*, rev. ed. (New Haven, CT: Yale University Press, 1989), p. 91.

6. Quoted in Veatch, *Death, Dying, and the Biological Revolution*, p. 91.

7. Jehovah's Witnesses are not opposed to blood substitutes, which can carry vast amounts of oxygen and do the work of blood until the patient's body has replenished its own supply. See *Time*, December 3, 1979, p. 90.

8. Veatch, *Death, Dying, and the Biological Revolution*, p. 92.

9. See Edward P. Richards III and Katharine C. Rathbun, *Law and the Physician* (Boston: Little, Brown, 1993), p. 171.

10. On this point, see Allen E. Buchanan and Dan W. Brock, *Deciding for Others* (New York: Cambridge University Press, 1989), Chapter 1, and Veatch, *Death, Dying, and the Biological Revolution*, p. 107.

11. See Veatch, *Death, Dying, and the Biological Revolution*, p. 129.

12. See Veatch, *Death, Dying, and the Biological Revolution*, p. 130.

13. Robert C. Underwood, "From *In re* Brooks Estate," in Samuel Gorovitz, Ruth Macklin, Andrew Jameton, John O'Connor, and Susan Sherwin (eds.), *Moral Problems in Medicine*, 2d ed. (Upper Saddle River, NJ: Prentice Hall, 1983), pp. 62–63.

14. Robert M. Veatch, *Case Studies in Medical Ethics* (Cambridge, MA: Harvard University Press, 1977), pp. 315–316.

15. See Veatch, *Death, Dying, and the Biological Revolution*, Chapter 5, especially pp. 117 and 131.

16. See Veatch, *Death, Dying, and the Biological Revolution*, pp. 132–133.

17. For extensive discussions of the Quinlan case, see Gregory E. Pence, *Classic Cases in Medical Ethics* (New York: McGraw-Hill, 1990), Chapter 1, and Veatch, *Death, Dying, and the Biological Revolution*, pp. 118–123.

18. See Pence, *Classic Cases in Medical Ethics*, pp. 7–13, and Veatch, *Death, Dying, and the Biological Revolution*, pp. 119–123.

19. For a discussion of cases of this sort, see Veatch, *Death, Dying, and the Biological Revolution*, pp. 134–136.

20. See Veatch, *Death, Dying, and the Biological Revolution*, pp. 133–134.

21. See *Guidelines on the Termination of Life-Sustaining Treatment and the Care of the Dying* (Bloomington: Indiana University Press, 1987), p. 66; Beauchamp and Childress, *Principles of Biomedical Ethics*, pp. 416–418; and M. D. Iseman, D. L. Cohn, and J. A. Sbarbaro, "Directly Observed Treatment of Tuberculosis: We Can't Afford Not to Try It," *New England Journal of Medicine*, Vol. 328 (1993), pp. 576–578.

22. See George J. Annas, "Forced Cesareans: The Most Unkindest Cut of All," *The Hastings Center Report*, Vol. 12 (June 1982), pp. 16–17, 45, and George J. Annas, *The Rights of Patients* (Totowa, NJ: Humana, 1992), pp. 128–130. Annas argues that the judges who ordered these cesarean sections made errors and that the law does not warrant such action.

23. See Veatch, *Death, Dying, and the Biological Revolution*, p. 98.

24. For a discussion of this case, see Pence, *Classic Cases in Medical Ethics*, Chapter 2, and Veatch, *Death, Dying, and the Biological Revolution*, pp. 89–91.

25. Pence, *Classic Cases in Medical Ethics*, p. 31.

26. See Veatch, *Death, Dying, and the Biological Revolution*, pp. 90, 100.

27. Late in 1985, Elizabeth Bouvia had another bout with the legal and medical establishments. She was a patient at High Desert Hospital (Los Angeles County, California). The hospital judged that her weight (between sixty-five and seventy pounds) was too little for her height (approximately five feet). They wanted to force-feed her for the purposes of increasing her weight. This time, with some complications, Bouvia won her legal battle. The issues in the two cases were different, however. This second time around Bouvia was not refusing nutrition and was not trying to starve herself. See Pence, *Classic Cases in Medical Ethics*, pp. 34ff.

28. Veatch, *Death, Dying, and the Biological Revolution*, pp. 104–105.

29. See Veatch, *Death, Dying, and the Biological Revolution*, p. 98.

30. One other exception not discussed here concerns prisoners, who are sometimes denied the right to refuse medical treatment. See Veatch, *Death, Dying, and the Biological Revolution*, pp. 105–106.

31. For a thorough explanation of the moral and legal issues involved in informed consent, see Ruth R. Faden and Tom L. Beauchamp, *A History and Theory of Informed Consent* (New York: Oxford University Press, 1986).

32. The five elements discussed here are explained in detail in Beauchamp and Childress, *Principles of Biomedical Ethics*, pp. 144–170.

33. For the relevance of cultural factors in related matters, see Benjamin Freedman, "Offering Truth," *Archives of Internal Medicine*, Vol. 153 (1993), pp. 572–576.

34. For an explanation of these cases, see Faden and Beauchamp, *A History and Theory of Informed Consent*, pp. 32–35, 132–138.

35. See Faden and Beauchamp, *A History and Theory of Informed Consent*, pp. 136–137.

36. See Faden and Beauchamp, *A History and Theory of Informed Consent*, pp. 38–39.

37. These codes are reprinted in the appendix.

38. Barbara Ridley, "Tom's Story: A Quadriplegic Who Refused Rehabilitation," *Rehabilitation Nursing*, Vol. 14 (Sept.–Oct. 1989), pp. 250–253.

39. Ruth Faden and Alan Faden, "False Belief and the Refusal of Medical Treatment," *Journal of Medical Ethics*, Vol. 3 (1977), pp. 133–136.

40. It should be pointed out that sociological factors complicated this case. The woman was a poor white from Appalachia with a third-grade education. The attending physician was black, which seemed to play a role in her refusal to believe his diagnosis. When a second (white) physician and her daughter became involved in the case, she finally consented to the hysterectomy. See Faden and Faden, "False Belief," p. 135.

41. See Veatch, *Death, Dying, and the Biological Revolution*, p. 105.

42. This distinction is explained in Gerasimos Santas, "The Socratic Paradoxes," *Philosophical Review*, Vol. 73 (1964), pp. 154–155.

43. See "A Demand to Die," in Bette-Jane Crigger (ed.), *Cases in Bioethics*, 2d ed. (New York: St. Martin's, 1993), pp. 118–122.

CHAPTER **4**

Euthanasia
and the Withdrawal
of Lifesaving Treatment

EUTHANASIA AND ABORTION, the topics in this and the next chapter, are sometimes called the life and death issues in medical ethics. Each of these issues has a social component and a private aspect. Because society has a legitimate interest in matters of life and death, it is appropriate for legislators to pass laws dealing with euthanasia and abortion. Yet individual health care practitioners must make decisions about these issues quite apart from what the law says. If a woman requests an abortion, the physician must decide whether to provide it. If a dying patient asks for a dosage of a lethal drug to hasten death, the health care professional must decide whether to comply with this request. And, difficult though this might be, it is possible that good morality and good law do not yield the same answers in every particular case.

One of the issues at stake in both euthanasia and abortion is the value of human life. Most will acknowledge that there is a prima facie duty to preserve human life. The interesting issue concerns when this duty may be overridden. Is it ever permissible not to preserve life? Is it ever permissible to hasten another's death? If so, when? Another issue raised in the debate about euthanasia is the extent to which we must honor a patient's autonomy. In the previous two chapters we have emphasized the value of autonomy and the rights of patients to control what happens to them in medical contexts. But if a patient explicitly requests measures to hasten death, must health care practitioners comply?

THE MORAL STATUS OF ACTIONS

Our principal concern here is with the permissibility of certain types of actions, in particular, actions designed to hasten the death of patients. So, as a preliminary matter, we must ask about the various moral statuses that actions might have.

Any given action might have one of at least three moral statuses.[1] Some actions are *morally required;* they are such that it would be morally wrong not to perform them. Keeping one's promises and telling the truth are acts that are normally morally required. The *morally neutral* constitutes a second moral category of actions. To say that an act is morally neutral is to say that the prospective agent may perform that act or may refrain from performing it; the agent is free to choose either course. Examples of morally neutral acts include your decision to wear your brown shoes, your decision to eat cereal for breakfast, and your decision to read Shakespeare last night. You might protest that these acts have nothing to do with morality, but that is just the point. This category, in which perhaps most of our actions fall, indicates that an action is neutral from the moral point of view. Actions that are required or neutral are also morally permissible; that is, agents are (at least) allowed to perform them. The third moral status that an action might have is that of being *morally forbidden.* An action that is morally forbidden is wrong to do. Uncontroversial examples of actions that are normally morally forbidden include killing, stealing, and torturing.

The moral status of actions is affected, in part, by the rights that beings have. Although we will not present a complete analysis of rights, we can at least review some of the points from the first chapter. Rights put legitimate moral restraints on how others may behave toward those who possess the rights. If a person has a right, then others have obligations with respect to that person. Positive and negative rights may be distinguished; the distinction is based on the sort of obligations that others have toward the rights holder. A *positive right* creates an obligation on someone else to perform a service or provide goods for the person possessing that right. For example, if Maria has promised to help Helga this afternoon, then Helga has a positive right against Maria. And Maria has an obligation to serve Helga in the manner promised. The rights of children to be fed, clothed, and nurtured by their parents are positive rights, rights that place obligations on the parents.

A *negative right,* by contrast, is a right to others' omissions or forbearances. For every negative right that a person possesses, someone else has an obligation to refrain from doing something. A person's property rights are usually understood as negative; they impose on others obligations not to use or deface another's property without the owner's permission. The right not to be tortured is also negative. How the right to life fits into this scheme will be addressed later.

TYPES OF EUTHANASIA

Dictionaries usually define *euthanasia* as a painless, easy death. In medical contexts, the term is used to designate an act designed to bring about such a death, usually in someone who is terminally ill. An act is not properly described as euthanasia unless at least two people are involved—a person whose death is induced and a person who plays a role in inducing that death—and unless the motive for the action is mercy or the good of the person whose death is hastened.

It is common to distinguish between active and passive euthanasia. *Active euthanasia* involves an act in which the death of a person is deliberately induced by doing something for that purpose when otherwise the person would continue living and where the agent's motive is mercy. It involves actively interfering with the natural course of events. It is mercy killing. *Passive euthanasia* is allowing death to come more quickly by stopping treatment or refraining from initiating treatment and where the agent's motive is mercy. It involves letting nature take its course. It is letting die rather than killing. Injecting a suffering patient with a lethal drug is active euthanasia; not employing CPR (cardiopulmonary resuscitation) when such a patient experiences cardiac or pulmonary arrest is passive euthanasia. Note that the difference between active and passive euthanasia is *not* whether physical action is involved. For withdrawing treatment is typically regarded as passive, though that involves an action. Presumably an important difference between active and passive euthanasia is the cause of death. With passive euthanasia, the disease process or medical condition is the cause of death; with active euthanasia, some element other than the patient's medical condition introduced by a second person is the cause of death.

The other important distinction is between voluntary and nonvoluntary euthanasia. Each of these can be coupled with either active or passive euthanasia, as the definitions will reveal. *Voluntary euthanasia* is either killing the patient or letting the patient die, where the agent's motive is mercy, only when the patient consents to or requests that this be done. *Nonvoluntary euthanasia* is either killing the patient or letting the patient die, where the agent's motive is mercy, when the patient has neither consented to nor requested that this be done. (Involuntary euthanasia is a special case of nonvoluntary, where the agent is acting *against* the patient's wishes. We shall not discuss involuntary euthanasia here.) In the typical cases of nonvoluntary euthanasia, patients are unable to make their own choices.

Given these two distinctions, four types of euthanasia are possible: (1) nonvoluntary active euthanasia, (2) nonvoluntary passive euthanasia, (3) voluntary active euthanasia, and (4) voluntary passive euthanasia. When discussing the morality of euthanasia and asking what the law should be regarding this practice, it is important to distinguish among these four possibilities. Most seem to agree that nonvoluntary active euthanasia is the most difficult to justify morally because it is killing a patient without his consent. And most seem to agree that voluntary passive euthanasia is the easiest to justify. Indeed, voluntary passive euthanasia is a special case of allowing a patient to refuse life-sustaining medical treatment. If euthanasia is passive, it involves withholding or withdrawing life-sustaining treatment; if it is voluntary, it is done in accord with the patient's wishes. It is a *special* case of permitting patients to refuse life-sustaining treatment because if it is genuinely euthanasia, then mercy is the principal motive for complying with the patient's wishes. This need not be the motive in other cases, such as when a Jehovah's Witness is permitted to refuse a blood transfusion. As we saw in the previous chapter, competent patients have the right to refuse medical treatment. So the topic of voluntary passive euthanasia need not detain us here.

Most agree that the distinction between voluntary and nonvoluntary euthanasia is morally important. It is easier to justify voluntary euthanasia because it involves no violation of autonomy. There is no such agreement, however, regarding the importance of the distinction between active and passive euthanasia. To be sure, the majority believe that this distinction is morally significant, but a vocal minority think that they are mistaken. Whether this latter distinction is important is our next topic.

ACTIVE AND PASSIVE EUTHANASIA

James Rachels is probably the best known among those who maintain that the distinction between active and passive euthanasia is of no moral importance.[2] Rachels assumes that the received view is that this distinction is crucial to assessing the morality of euthanasia. Such a view even seems to have received official endorsement from the House of Delegates of the American Medical Association on December 4, 1973:

> The intentional termination of the life of one human being by another—mercy killing—is contrary to that for which the medical profession stands and is contrary to the policy of the American Medical Association.
>
> The cessation of the employment of extraordinary means to prolong the life of the body when there is irrefutable evidence that biological death is imminent is the decision of the patient and/or his immediate family. The advice and judgment of the physician should be freely available to the patient and/or his immediate family.

Rachels believes that in this statement, the AMA is committed to two claims: (1) there is a morally relevant difference between active and passive euthanasia, and (2) that difference is such that active euthanasia is never permissible, but voluntary passive euthanasia is permissible if death is imminent. Rachels wants to convince readers that there is usually no moral difference between active and passive euthanasia, and, when there is a difference, passive euthanasia is not always morally preferable. Rachels makes a number of points, but we will discuss just four in particular here.

Rachels's first point is that in many cases, active euthanasia is more humane than passive euthanasia. Examples illustrate this claim. Consider the plight of the patient with terminal and incurable throat cancer. Suppose that he will die within a few weeks even if treatment is continued but that he does not want to continue suffering. If the physician agrees to withhold treatment, it still may take a long time for the patient to die, and during that period his suffering may be difficult to control. Rachels contends that once the decision has been made not to prolong a patient's agony, active euthanasia is preferable to passive euthanasia because passive euthanasia allows the suffering to continue, perhaps for a longer time than is predicted.

Rachels's second criticism of the conventional doctrine embodied in the AMA statement is this: it leads to decisions regarding life and death that are made on irrelevant grounds. He asks us to consider the case of a Down's syndrome infant who also has an intestinal obstruction. This obstruction must be corrected surgically for the infant to live. Rachels points out that parents have sometimes been permitted to decline such lifesaving surgery. The reason that parents refuse such surgery, of course, is that the child has Down's syndrome and the parents do not want her to live. But Rachels argues that this is absurd. If the life of such an infant is worth preserving, what difference does it make if it needs a simple operation? And if one thinks that the baby should not live, what difference does it make if it happens to have an obstructed intestinal tract? Rachels's point is that if the infant had Down's syndrome but no life-threatening intestinal blockage, it would be allowed to live. And if it had an intestinal blockage but no Down's syndrome, it would be allowed to live. But surely the fact that it has both Down's syndrome and a blocked intestine is an accident that has no moral significance. Yet, Rachels thinks, people are so obsessed with the conventional view that they think it is permissible to let such infants die; exercising such an option is merely passive euthanasia.

Rachels's third criticism is that the AMA statement rests on a distinction between killing and letting die that itself has no moral significance. To convince you of this, Rachels discusses the parallel cases of Jones and Smith. These two cases are designed to be alike in all respects except one: one involves killing; the other, letting die. Jones and Smith each will benefit financially from the death of his respective six-year-old cousin. Each concocts a plan to drown his cousin in the bathtub and make it look like an accident. Jones executes his plan and kills his cousin. Smith sets out to do the same thing. But as Smith enters the bathroom, his cousin slips, hits his head, and is rendered unconscious. Smith considers himself lucky: now he does not have to kill his cousin but merely let him die. Rachels says that there is no morally relevant difference between the behavior of Jones and of Smith; each is equally reprehensible. Of course, cases of euthanasia are not like this. Doctors do not kill patients or let them die for personal gain. But Rachels's point is that the bare difference between killing and letting die does not itself make a moral difference.

Some argue that the important difference between active and passive euthanasia is this: in passive euthanasia, the physician does not do anything to bring about the patient's death; in active euthanasia, the physician does something to bring about the patient's death. Because agents are more responsible for their acts than their omissions, active euthanasia is more serious than passive euthanasia. But Rachels thinks that this view is mistaken, leading to his fourth criticism of the conventional view. The mistake is to regard omissions as doing nothing and to assume that agents are less responsible for omissions than for actions. If a physician could save a patient's life by giving her medication but decides not to do so, it is not true that the physician did nothing; the physician let the patient die and is responsible for so doing. To say that one is always more responsible for one's acts than for one's omissions is, therefore, false.

In making these four criticisms, Rachels's overall point is not to defend active euthanasia, though he does favor it in certain situations. Rather, his point is that the mere difference between active and passive euthanasia has no *moral* relevance. If the situation is the same, then if passive euthanasia is permissible, active euthanasia should be permissible too. If the patient's death is a good thing, then either type of euthanasia leads to that end. And if active euthanasia is wrong in a given case, then passive euthanasia should be wrong too. If death is undesirable, it should not matter what means is employed to achieve it. Rachels recognizes that *the law* prohibits active euthanasia and sometimes permits passive euthanasia, and health care practitioners may have to take this into account. But his point is that this position embodied in the law is morally indefensible. And in the AMA statement, physicians appear to be agreeing with the law.

Not all of Rachels's criticisms of the conventional view are convincing. His second objection is surely mistaken. We have no reason to believe that the conventional view or the AMA statement would approve of withholding the lifesaving treatment from the Down's syndrome infant. Indeed, there is reason to believe that they would disapprove of withholding the surgery; death is not imminent and the treatment is not extraordinary. Perhaps Rachels's point is simply that the emphasis on the difference between active and passive euthanasia has led society to approve of too many instances of letting die. This may be true, but the AMA statement does not endorse the practice that Rachels condemns.

Rachels's memorable examples of Jones and Smith miss the point. From these parallel cases, Rachels seems to conclude that there is never a morally relevant difference between killing and letting die. But they do not establish this. In Rachels's two parallel cases, killing and letting die are *both wrong*. But there is nothing in the AMA statement to preclude this possibility. The AMA statement *disapproves* of *all* cases of killing, but it does *not approve* of *all* cases of letting die. A defender of the AMA statement can consistently agree with Rachels that both Jones and Smith did wrong. There is a pair of parallel cases that would refute the AMA statement, but it is different from that offered by Rachels. The parallel pair needed to do the job is this: a case in which letting a patient die is permissible according to the AMA statement, and a case exactly like that in all respects except that it involves killing—and most people would agree that killing in this situation is permissible. This is the combination that the AMA statement precludes. If one is to employ Rachels's strategy for refutation, one must come up with parallel cases of this sort.

Some, including Bonnie Steinbock, think that Rachels has completely misunderstood what the AMA statement says.[3] According to Steinbock, what the AMA statement condemns is the intentional termination of life, and so it rejects *both* active and passive euthanasia. The AMA statement does permit the cessation of life-sustaining treatment in certain situations, but it is a mistake to think that position is tantamount to endorsing passive euthanasia. Steinbock maintains that with both active and passive euthanasia, the object is to hasten the patient's death; the means of achieving the end are just different. Nevertheless, each involves the intentional termination of life, which the AMA statement forbids.

At this point, you might protest that the cessation of life-sustaining treatment also has as its point the patient's death. After all, health care practitioners who withhold or withdraw such treatment know that the patient will die as a result. So is that not their object? Steinbock's answer is that it need not be. In at least two situations the cessation of life-sustaining treatment is *not* the intentional termination of the life of one human being by another. The first is when a competent patient exercises his right to refuse treatment. Here the point of stopping treatment is not to bring about the patient's death; rather, it is to honor the patient's right to self-determination. The second of these situations occurs when the treatment in question has little or no chance of benefiting the patient. The point of withdrawing treatment in this type of case is that it is not helping the patient; it may even be harming the patient, depending on its degree of invasiveness. If this view is correct, it tells us that the proper way to understand what is meant by "extraordinary" treatment is treatment that will not, on balance, help the patient. As a result, whether any given treatment is extraordinary depends on the circumstances and whether it is likely to provide the patient with more benefits than burdens.[4]

We cannot here resolve the issue of whether Rachels's attack on the moral relevance of the distinction between active and passive euthanasia is successful. Rachels's most important challenge is his contention that in some cases active euthanasia is more humane than passive euthanasia; this point is especially important because mercy is the most creditable motive in cases of euthanasia. If this is correct, something is unsettling about our society's penchant to approve of only passive euthanasia. Another doctrine, however, may provide a basis for something akin to the conventional view.

THE DOCTRINE OF DOUBLE EFFECT

The doctrine of double effect is based on a distinction between what a person foresees will result from her action and what a person intends by such action. What is it that a person intends when she performs a voluntary action? According to this doctrine, a person *intends* in the strictest sense only those things that she *aims at as ends* or *as direct means* to such ends. A consequence of an action that a person knows will occur but that is neither the end sought nor the direct means to the end is said to be merely *foreseen*.

To understand this distinction, consider an example. A patient has a serious form of cancer. This patient's physician recommends chemotherapy. The physician realizes that as a result of this treatment, the patient will become nauseous and experience hair loss, among other things. The end that this physician is aiming at is to do what is best for this patient. The means to this end is to initiate a regimen of chemotherapy. A foreseen but unintended consequence is that the patient will become nauseous and lose hair. This result is unintended because it is neither the end sought nor the direct means to that end. It makes sense to say that this consequence is unintended because the physician in no way desires this end; if it were possible to administer chemotherapy without the accompanying nausea and hair loss, the physician would do so.

According to the doctrine of double effect, agents are more responsible for what is intended as a result of their voluntary actions than for merely what is foreseen will follow from such actions. Given these distinctions, the doctrine of double effect may now be stated as follows: It is permissible to bring about through voluntary actions an evil state of affairs just in case (1) the agent does not intend the evil that results, and (2) performing the action prevents a greater evil or the evil that does occur could only be prevented if the agent were to do evil intentionally.

To explain the doctrine briefly, clause 1 states that it is never permissible for an agent, through voluntary actions, to bring about evil if that evil is the end sought or a direct means to that end. Clause 2 invokes a kind of proportionality. It states that even when an evil (bad) state of affairs brought about is foreseen but unintended, it is permissible to allow it to occur only if doing so prevents a greater evil or is the only alternative to doing evil intentionally. The principle is called the doctrine of double effect because it distinguishes, for moral reasons, two different effects of an action: those aimed at or intended and those foreseen but in no way desired. (The doctrine says nothing about a third type of effect, namely, unforeseen consequences. Presumably it holds that these are morally irrelevant unless the agent is negligent.) The doctrine of double effect forbids a person to do evil intentionally. Bringing about a bad state of affairs is permitted only when the agent does not intend this.

Why should anyone accept this doctrine? One reason for doing so is that it yields plausible judgments in particular cases. For example, health care practitioners sometimes provide large quantities of narcotic analgesics to dying patients to relieve their suffering. Doing this, however, can lead to respiratory depression in these patients, thereby hastening their deaths. In spite of this result, administering the narcotics seems right, and the doctrine of double effect explains why this practice is not wrongful killing. The end is to relieve suffering, and administering narcotics is the means to that end. That the patient's death is hastened is a foreseen but unintended consequence.[5]

The doctrine of double effect also supports Steinbock's reading of the AMA statement and supports a position that many health care professionals believe. Many do not want to prohibit withdrawing life-sustaining treatment when the patient requests it or administering narcotics to relieve the patient's suffering even if it hastens death. But they do want to prohibit physician-assisted suicide and active euthanasia.[6] Since the latter two practices aim at the patient's death, they are forbidden by the doctrine of double effect. But the former activities are not so prohibited.

Is the doctrine of double effect a plausible view? One criticism, suggested by James Rachels,[7] says that the doctrine of double effect incorrectly implies that an agent's intention is relevant to the rightness or wrongness of that agent's act. To convince you that it is not relevant, Rachels offers examples. Imagine that Jack visits his sick grandmother for the afternoon. His only intention is to cheer her up; he is aware that this could influence the writing of her will, but he has no such motive. Jill also visits her grandmother, but her only concern is to influence the will. Both Jack and Jill succeed in cheering up their grandmothers. Rachels says that either both did what is right, or both did what is wrong. After all, each did the same thing—bring cheer to a grandmother. The agent's intention has nothing to do with the rightness or wrongness of his behavior. The moral relevance of intentions concerns the agent's *character*, not actions. Thus, we might say that Jack is admirable and Jill is not. But their actions can be assessed without referring to those character traits. In fairness to defenders of the doctrine of double effect, however, we should note that Rachels seems to assume the controversial view that the only morally relevant feature of actions is their consequences.

The doctrine of double effect gives rise to other suspicions. The distinction between what is intended and what is merely foreseen sometimes seems blurry, which generates the following criticism: Through verbal manipulation, a sufficiently clever person can justify almost any action by using the doctrine of double effect.[8] To illustrate this, the following familiar case is sometimes cited. A group of ten people are exploring in a cave near the ocean. As they ascend from the cave, their leader becomes stuck in the entrance. The waters are rising rapidly; if the man is not freed from the entrance, the others will drown. A member of the group happens to have some explosives. Now the nine spelunkers have two choices. They can use the explosives on the one who is trapped, thereby killing one but saving nine; or they can do nothing, thereby allowing one to live and nine to die. Now imagine that one of nine uses the doctrine of double effect and reasons as follows:

> We are permitted to save the nine. The end of our act is to save nine people. The direct means to that end is to widen the entrance to the cave. A foreseen but unintended consequence is that the man will be killed. But since the death of the man is neither the end sought nor the direct means to that end and since his death prevents a greater evil, we are permitted to do that which brings about his death.

The criticism of this reasoning is *not* that it inappropriately permits the killing of the one to save the nine. This is a very difficult case, and killing the trapped man may be permissible. The criticism concerns the way in which this conclusion is justified. It seems to involve verbal manipulation. Describing the means to be employed as "widening the entrance" and the foreseen but unintended consequence as "the man will be killed" seems disingenuous. If a doctrine permits such sophistry, that is an argument against it. A sufficiently clever person could justify any conclusion by analogous reasoning, and, if so, the doctrine of double effect is unacceptable.

We leave unresolved for now the issues of whether the AMA statement can be defended, whether the doctrine of double effect should be rejected, and whether active euthanasia is always wrong. Our next topic concerns the legalization of euthanasia.

LEGALIZING EUTHANASIA

Much debate continues concerning the legalization of euthanasia. Many different pieces of euthanasia legislation have been proposed. Here we shall indicate what sort of questions need to be answered before we can adequately assess any given proposal. Then we shall discuss arguments for and against legalizing euthanasia.

Four Questions

To evaluate any proposed piece of legislation concerning euthanasia, we must address four questions. (1) Under the proposal in question, who are the possible subjects or candidates for euthanasia? That is, if the legislative proposal were adopted, whom would it be permissible to euthanize? (2) Does the proposal allow only for voluntary euthanasia, or does it also allow for nonvoluntary euthanasia? (3) Does the proposal allow for both active and passive euthanasia, or does it permit only passive? (4) What safeguards are built into the legislation to protect against the possibility of abuse? Each of these questions will be discussed.

Question 1 Different legislative proposals include different groups as possible subjects. To identify with the issue here, ask yourself, "Under what conditions would I want euthanasia for myself?" Several categories are possible here; the five most commonly cited will be discussed briefly.

First, many say that if they had a painful and terminal illness, such as throat cancer, they would choose euthanasia for themselves if that were an option. These are patients who will die soon anyway and who will be in great pain until death. Proponents say that not allowing such patients to hasten their deaths forces them to suffer for no reason. With this group of subjects, the goal is to minimize human suffering.

Second, some say that if they were permanently unconscious or in a persistent vegetative state, they would not want to be kept alive. Though the continued existence of these individuals is not painful for them, they believe that it is meaningless. Usually such patients are being kept alive by various medical interventions, including artificial feeding, respirators, and the like. And sometimes these patients live for a long time. Probably no case in medical ethics has received more publicity than that of Karen Quinlan (discussed in Chapter 3). As a result of this case, many people fear ending their lives in this way, which in part accounts for the strong feelings that many have about the inclusion of the second category.

Third, some say that severely deformed infants are beings on whom it should be permissible to practice euthanasia. What people have in mind here are infants whose severe abnormalities cause them great pain or make living impossible. Clearly, anencephalic infants (ones born without a brain) qualify here; though they do not suffer, they will never be conscious. Listing other categories confidently is difficult because any given condition can vary greatly in its severity. The idea is to focus on the prospects of the individual infant, and euthanasia is a viable option only for those whose prospects are horrible.

Fourth, some say that they would want to opt for euthanasia for themselves if they were suffering from severe senility, such as Alzheimer's disease. This category is not included because of suffering, though in fact many such patients do experience considerable frustration. But many who fear living this way focus instead on what they regard as the undignified state of such existence. When people talk about "death with dignity," they usually have in mind the undignified states of persons in the second and fourth categories.

Some expand the list to include a fifth category. It is more difficult to label, but it includes persons who have permanently lost things of greatest value to them. An example is provided from the movie *Whose Life Is It, Anyway?* The protagonist is a sculptor and university professor. His life, which has revolved around his work and girlfriend, is dramatically altered when he is in a serious automobile accident. The accident causes paralysis from the neck down and serious kidney damage. Because of the latter, the patient needs dialysis. After several months, he asks his physician if the paralysis is permanent. He receives the answer that he has suspected; he will be a quadriplegic for life. He does not want to live this way. Being unable to continue his work and normal activities with his girlfriend is more than he can handle. He asks that dialysis be stopped, knowing that this will result in his death. Of course, this case is essentially one of a competent patient requesting that treatment be discontinued. But it does illustrate how the issues of treatment refusal and euthanasia can come together.

Question 2   Most proposed pieces of legislation allow only for voluntary euthanasia. Some question arises, however, about what cases may be included under the description "voluntary euthanasia." Usually euthanasia is considered voluntary only if the consent of the person whose life is ended is obtained. But exactly what counts as genuine consent here?

There are several possibilities. One notion of voluntary euthanasia is very narrow; consent is genuine only if the person has requested here and now that the act take place. This account is narrow because unless a person is able to and does make her request known at the time the act is desired, consent has not been given and euthanasia cannot be voluntary.

A second notion of voluntary euthanasia is broader in that it allows for persons to consent by stating their wishes in advance. Persons may specify that if certain conditions obtain they do not wish to be kept alive. Documents known as "living wills" and "advanced directives" enable people to convey their wishes in this way. According to this second account, if people have properly executed such a document, then any act of euthanasia in accord with their wishes is voluntary. Only competent persons can execute such documents.

A third and even broader notion not only counts an act as voluntary euthanasia if the patient's consent has been given (either here and now or in advance) but also allows for proxy consent. *Proxy consent* occurs when one person consents on behalf of another. The person or persons legally authorized to speak for you might give consent. The authorized person may be your spouse, grown children, parents, or siblings, usually in that order. Proxy consent is not in any literal sense a person's own choice. But it might be assumed that a spouse, child, parent, or sibling knows the patient's wishes and will act to see that they are fulfilled.

Proxy consent should not be confused with a *health care power of attorney*. To explain the latter, in most states you can designate someone as your health care agent. If you have done so, then when you are not competent, the person you have designated is authorized to make your health care decisions. Health care agents can make only medical decisions; they do not have the broader power of attorney. In some states, a health care agent's decision-making powers are limited; in others, the agent has the same authority that the patient has when competent, unless the patient has explicitly limited the agent's powers.

If following the instructions of a health care agent counts as voluntary, it falls under the second of the three notions described earlier. In designating someone as your health care agent, you have determined who will make your medical decisions. This act is not the same as devising a living will or advanced directive, where you try to determine what specific decisions will be made. But by designating someone as your health care agent, you authorize that person to make your medical decisions when you are not competent. With proxy consent, the law determines who may speak for you, typically based on kinship.

It is important to realize that how the notion of consent is interpreted is not merely a verbal dispute. For understandable reasons, few are willing to advocate nonvoluntary euthanasia. But if cases of legally permitted euthanasia are limited to those in which consent is present, then we must be absolutely clear about what counts as consent. And notice the practical implications. Suppose that we adopt the narrow understanding of voluntary euthanasia: euthanasia is voluntary only if the patient has consented here and now. Of the five types of cases mentioned where euthanasia might be desirable, only the first and fifth can count as voluntary in this narrow sense. For only in these two cases can the patient be competent at the time of the act. Clearly persons suffering from severe senility, persons who are unconscious, and infants are not competent. And even in the first case—persons suffering from a terminal, painful illness—competence may be questioned if the pain is all-consuming. So to adopt the narrow account is to allow for very few cases of euthanasia, at least when it is restricted to voluntary euthanasia.

If we adopt the second account and count as voluntary cases in which consent is given in advance, then this will allow for euthanasia in *some* of the cases in which the patient is severely senile and in *some* of the cases in which the patient is permanently unconscious—namely, when the patients have properly executed the relevant legal document. But this view could not include persons who lapsed into permanent unconsciousness before attaining legal competence. And it could not include any severely deformed infants. Indeed, any sort of euthanasia for severely deformed infants or persons who lapsed into permanent unconsciousness before attaining competence can be voluntary only if the third sense of that term is employed. But to count proxy consent as voluntary is surely to misuse that term. Someone else's consenting to euthanasia for you does not make your death voluntary. One suspects that those who use the term *voluntary* in this third sense believe that some sort of euthanasia is justifiable in certain cases involving infants or minors, but they are unwilling to approve of nonvoluntary euthanasia. To stretch the term *voluntary* in this way is to lose the moral point of the original distinction.

Question 3 This question asks whether a proposed statute allows for active euthanasia or only for passive euthanasia. As noted earlier, in both the medical and legal communities, active euthanasia is widely condemned, and certain instances of passive euthanasia are acceptable. Active euthanasia is typically regarded as homicide and said always to be wrong. Notice, however, the consequences of limiting legally permitted acts of euthanasia to the passive cases only. Many cases where people believe that euthanasia is desirable will be cases where its point cannot be achieved unless its active form is practiced.

Consider again the case of a person suffering from a painful, terminal illness. If euthanasia is desirable here, its purpose is to relieve needless suffering. But this goal is best achieved through active euthanasia; for if passive euthanasia is the only option and treatment is merely stopped, the patient's dying process and suffering may drag on for a long time. And in some cases where the patient is permanently unconscious (and so not suffering), stopping treatment does not always end what the patient herself would have regarded as an undignified existence—as the case of Karen Quinlan reminds us.

Before turning to the final question, two points should be made. First, if we restrict euthanasia to voluntary passive euthanasia and we understand "voluntary" in the narrowest sense, only one of the five categories of candidates for euthanasia identified earlier is eligible. Patients in the first category—those suffering from painful, terminal illnesses—could not relieve the needless suffering with only passive euthanasia. Those in the second, third, and fourth categories are not competent at the time the act (or omission) is to be performed and so cannot consent in the relevant sense. Only some of those in the fifth category will be eligible.

This consideration is one reason that crafting legislation regarding euthanasia is difficult. The kind of cases that legislators would like to capture do not match people's beliefs about the more abstract distinctions. Second, the term *passive euthanasia* is seldom used today. As a result, many people have come to identify *euthanasia* with active euthanasia. Passive euthanasia is simply thought of as withholding or withdrawing life-extending treatment, and the controversial term *euthanasia* has been dropped in these cases. You should keep this in mind when reading discussions of this topic in newspapers and magazines.

Question 4 What safeguards are built into the legislation to protect against the possibility of abuse? The worry here is that if one human being is allowed to hasten the death of another, things may get out of hand. Many safeguards have been proposed by those who favor enacting euthanasia legislation, but only a few will be mentioned here.[9]

One common safeguard is to restrict euthanasia to those who themselves have requested the act. A second safeguard is to require that patients be legally competent to make their own decisions. This step is designed to prevent those who are too immature from making such an irreversible decision. Third, many require that the agent of the act be a physician who has consulted with at least one other physician. This precaution is designed to minimize medical errors. Before engaging in euthanasia, physicians must be as sure as they can be that the case is hopeless. The requirement that the agent be a physician is apparently paternalistic, and perhaps justifiable. If anyone were permitted to engage in euthanasia, patients temporarily in pain may ask others with no medical knowledge to assist in hastening their deaths. Persons with medical expertise may refuse, however, because they know that this condition is only temporary. The person's request is irrational, but only a qualified health care professional is apt to know this. Fourth, some require that the patient must have no doubts and must have repeated the request several times. Finally, some suggest that a certain period of time must elapse between the request and the act itself. This measure is designed to ensure that the patient really wants to die; it allows for changes of mind at the last minute. This safeguard appears to be based on weak paternalism.

If we ask these four questions at the outset, we will be better positioned to evaluate any given piece of legislation regarding euthanasia. We will have a framework for understanding the proposal.

Pros and Cons

Let us now ask what sort of reasons have been given to support the claim that euthanasia should be legally permissible. Proponents have contended that voluntary euthanasia promotes two widely shared values. First, it is desirable to prevent needless suffering. Persons who are terminally ill, in great pain, and request that death be hastened are suffering for no good purpose. Euthanasia promotes beneficence in these cases.

Liberty or personal autonomy is the second value that voluntary euthanasia promotes. People should be allowed to make their own choices and
control their own destinies; we should interfere with them only when
they inflict harm on nonconsenting parties. So, the argument goes, we
should not prohibit *voluntary* euthanasia.

A third reason sometimes given in support of voluntary euthanasia is
that it promotes "death with dignity." It is not easy to explain what this is
or how exactly it is related to beneficence or autonomy, but we have some
idea of what proponents have in mind here. They point to examples
where death is decidedly not dignified, such as in the case of Karen
Quinlan. When people say that they would not want to be maintained the
way that Quinlan was, presumably they understand that she was not in
pain; what they fear is the undignified state. Some may call such a fear
irrational, since individuals in such a state have no experiences and so are
unaware of what is happening. But to so label this common fear seems
unwarranted; for people care not only about what they experience but
also about how others remember them.

Not everyone supports the legalization of euthanasia. The case
against nonvoluntary euthanasia is the clearest and most convincing.
Such an act, without consent, deprives persons of their right to life and is
also a violation of personal autonomy. Whether people may justifiably
decide to end their own lives is arguable, but surely others may not normally make this decision. And one suspects that the possibilities of abuse
are much greater in the case of nonvoluntary euthanasia.

But why have people objected to the legalization of voluntary euthanasia? Why is it wrong for a society to allow its citizens to choose assisted
death for themselves in these extreme cases? Many objections have been
raised against legalizing even voluntary euthanasia, and some of these
will be discussed here. Replies to these objections will also be explained.

The first objection is frequently articulated by those associated with
the hospice movement.[10] They argue that the humanitarian goal of preventing suffering can be achieved without deliberately hastening the
patient's death. Modern techniques for controlling pain should be employed so that patients can be kept alive and comfortable for as long as
possible. They claim that physicians in the United States have done a very
poor job of relieving pain and that they have much to learn from their
European counterparts.

The second objection begins with the assertion that it is often difficult
to determine whether a person has genuinely consented to euthanasia.
The critics' point is that what appear to be cases of voluntary euthanasia
may not be that at all. They support this criticism with several claims. If
consent is given during the final stages of a painful illness, during mo-

ments of great pain or under the influence of heavy sedation, the patient's capability of giving informed consent will be doubted. If the person has given consent in advance, such as in a living will, we cannot be sure whether he has had a change of mind. Even if that doubt were eradicated, living wills are so vague that it will be difficult to tell whether the patient's current condition matches those conditions specified in that document. And if the patient's wishes have been conveyed only verbally, matters may be even more difficult. Karen Quinlan, when competent, allegedly expressed to others the wish not to be maintained artificially if there were no hope for recovery. But was she serious when she said this? Had she given the matter much thought? Would she have wanted artificial nutrition stopped? In addition, some worry that a patient will "consent" to euthanasia to relieve relatives or family members of their suffering. This reaction is akin to succumbing to pressure, they say.

Even if we could determine with certainty that consent was genuine, it would not be enough. For, according to critics, the facts that the victim consents and that the actor's motives are humanitarian provide no legal or moral defense for killing. This is the third objection to legalizing voluntary euthanasia. In our legal system, if a person walks up to you and asks you to kill her, you are not justified in doing so. According to the critic, voluntary euthanasia is no different from this case.

This objection rests on the assumption that the right to life is inalienable. A right is *inalienable* if it may not be waived or transferred by its possessor; a right is *alienable* if it may be waived or transferred by its possessor. Property rights are uncontroversially alienable. Since you purchased this book, you have property rights to it. You may give this book to a friend; in so doing, you have transferred certain property rights to that person. You also have property rights to the land that you purchased. You may, however, waive some of those rights and allow me to walk across it daily to arrive at my destination more quickly. But, according to the critic, not all rights are like this. Some rights, including the right to life, are inalienable, and so the possessor may not give others permission to infringe that right. As a result, even *voluntary* euthanasia should be proscribed.

The fourth objection to legalizing voluntary euthanasia is presented in the form of a dilemma. It concerns the desirability of including safeguards in any statute permitting euthanasia. Critics claim that if all of the appropriate restrictions are included in the legislation, then very few people will benefit and the main purposes of euthanasia will have been lost. Several points are cited to establish this horn of the dilemma: if we permit only voluntary euthanasia, many persons who are permanently unconscious will not qualify; if only passive euthanasia is permitted, then we will be unable to prevent much of the suffering experienced by those with painful, terminal illnesses; and if a time lapse is required between the request and the act, additional suffering will occur. On the other hand, if such safeguards are not included in the law, then the possibilities of abuse by relatives, health care practitioners, and others are too great. Surely most will agree that the conditions under which one human being is allowed to end the life of another must be carefully regulated. As a result, proponents of legalizing voluntary euthanasia face a dilemma.

The choice to have one's life ended, if carried out, is irrevocable, which gives rise to the fifth objection. According to critics, people should avoid making irrevocable decisions whenever possible. A canon of rationality states that people should keep as many options open to themselves for as long as possible. But the choice of euthanasia, if exercised, is not only irreversible; it also forecloses all other options. So, people should not be permitted to make such choices.

The sixth objection, closely related to the fifth, asserts that the judgment that a person is terminally ill may be mistaken in either of two ways. First, a diagnostic error is always possible. Physicians may judge that patients have terminal illnesses when in fact they do not. If a physician consults with another doctor, the possibility of such an error is lessened; but a possibility still exists. Second, a new cure may be discovered for the illness after the patient has been euthanized but before that patient would have died of natural causes. Thus, contrary to the physician's belief, the patient could have been saved.

The seventh and final objection to be discussed here is also the most important. It is the so-called *wedge argument,* also called the *slippery slope argument.* This argument has two versions, each of which takes the following form: "If we accept X, then Y follows, and Y is undesirable." The two versions of the argument differ regarding the interpretation of "follows."[11] According to the *logical* version of the wedge argument, Y follows logically from X; that is, if we accept X, then logically we must accept Y. And if Y is false or undesirable, that is a good reason not to accept X. The logical version of the wedge argument was employed at the end of Chapter 3 in criticizing the rationale to justify some cases of treatment without consent.

When criticizing the legalization of voluntary euthanasia, however, usually the *empirical* version of the wedge argument is advanced. According to this view, Y follows from X, not as a logical consequence but as a likely *causal consequence.* As applied to the legalization of voluntary euthanasia, the empirical version of the wedge argument says that we must examine the probable impact of changing laws and making exceptions to rules. It claims that if any of the stringent restraints against killing other human beings is removed, a moral decline is likely to follow. Because of various psychological and social factors, it is unlikely that people will draw distinctions that are clear and defensible. To authorize killing patients for their own benefit when they are suffering great pain or have bleak futures can easily open the door to killing patients for social benefits, such as reducing financial burdens. And it is all too easy to move from voluntary to nonvoluntary euthanasia. Again, because it would be convenient for society to rid itself of certain individuals whose care is quite expensive, people will stretch the notion of what counts as consenting to one's own death far beyond what is currently recognized.

Advocates of the causal version of the wedge argument say that even if there are clear *logical distinctions* between a patient's benefit and social benefit, and between voluntary and nonvoluntary euthanasia, the presence of other social factors—such as limited resources, large numbers of newborns with disabilities, many aged persons with serious illnesses, racism, and the like—will lead people to stretch otherwise reasonable principles beyond their logical bounds. So, as a result of taking the step of legalizing voluntary euthanasia, society will be led to practices that most agree are unacceptable. The only way to avoid this is not to take that step.

Proponents of legalizing voluntary euthanasia have not been convinced by these objections. Although we cannot deal here with each objection in detail, let us indicate briefly how proponents respond. Readers can develop these brief suggestions further as they see fit.

In response to the first objection, many acknowledge that in the United States physicians have not done a very good job of managing patients' pain; on this count, they have much to learn from others. But proponents of legalizing voluntary euthanasia say that only in *some* cases can suffering be relieved without hastening the patient's death; in others, death provides the only relief. Moreover, this objection ignores the fact that patients may fear dependence and what they perceive as an undignified existence as well as pain, particularly with progressive and debilitating diseases such as Huntington's chorea and amyotrophic lateral sclerosis (commonly known as Lou Gehrig's disease), or dementia often associated with the final stages of AIDS.[12]

According to the second objection, many factors make it difficult to determine whether a patient's consent is genuine. In general, proponents of legalizing voluntary euthanasia say it is based on exaggerated claims. They acknowledge that in some cases it is hard to ascertain whether consent is genuine; but on the whole, extreme skepticism is not warranted about these matters. Experienced health care professionals can usually tell when consent is genuine; and when in doubt, they can err on the side of life.

The third objection holds that the patient's consent does not justify hastening his death because the right to life is inalienable. One possible response here is to deny that the right to life is inalienable. If one is not inclined to try to tangle with the traditional view of the right to life, however, one might instead argue that the inalienability of this right does not preclude the permissibility of voluntary euthanasia.[13] One might argue, for example, that though the possessor's consent alone does not justify killing, consent in combination with other relevant conditions, such as the presence of a painful, terminal illness, does justify such an act. If this line can be developed, the third objection can be answered.

To the fourth objection, the dilemma, defenders of voluntary euthanasia respond that even if it is true that only a few will benefit when the necessary safeguards are included, that is not a good reason to delay the legislation. If even a few can be spared unnecessary pain, that is a good thing. Moreover, proponents doubt that only a few will benefit from such legislation; they believe that their opponents are exaggerating.

One cannot deny that the decision to have one's life ended, if carried out, is irrevocable. But opponents of voluntary euthanasia assume that people should avoid making irrevocable decisions whenever possible, and that assumption is dubious. It is more plausible to say that one should be very careful before making such decisions. Consider a related matter. Marriage is not irrevocable, but it is typically (emotionally) painful to revoke. It does not follow that one should always avoid getting married; but the wise person will not enter marriage without considerable thought. Perhaps an even better example is the decision to have children. Once the deed is done, one cannot cease to be a biological parent. And given the enormous responsibilities associated with that role, such a decision should not be entered into lightly. Yet it is not irrational to decide to have children.

One part of the sixth objection says that the physician's diagnosis may be mistaken and euthanasia in such cases would be a tragic mistake. One cannot deny that physicians make diagnostic errors. But proponents of voluntary euthanasia advocate regulation designed to minimize such mistakes. If euthanasia is permitted only for those with certain medical conditions, and if the presence of that condition must be confirmed by a second, independent physician, these steps will minimize errors. Even with consultation, obviously errors can occur. But defenders of voluntary euthanasia say that the issue is the overall good of society. Denying relief from suffering is unfair to many because of the possibility of rare diagnostic errors. And since we are talking about *voluntary* euthanasia, patients themselves are aware of possible mistakes and may take that into account in making decisions.

The other part of this objection says that a new cure may be discovered tomorrow. For the most part, this opinion is based on a naive, unrealistic picture of medical discovery. The critics seem to think that a scientific breakthrough made today will result in the mass production of a miracle cure tomorrow. But discovery in medical contexts typically does not work this way. After initial breakthroughs, much testing is required before drugs or treatments may be used routinely on human beings. Years may elapse before a treatment is made available to the general public. Assuming that physicians keep up with the current research in their fields, they will know whether promising breakthroughs have occurred and will so inform their patients. Holding out for a miracle cure when no progress has been made is unrealistic.

A full discussion of the wedge argument is not possible here. Defenders of voluntary euthanasia have made several points in reply. First, they claim that if the safeguards mentioned earlier are included, the likelihood of abuses will decrease. Second, they try to shift the burden of proof to their critics. They accuse the critics of employing scare tactics and ask what specific evidence they can provide to show that these terrible consequences will ensue if only voluntary euthanasia is legalized. Empirical evidence is needed here. Perhaps it would be helpful to study the situation in the Netherlands, where voluntary active euthanasia has been allowed but not formally legalized.[14] Even here, though, some wonder whether other cultural differences will make such a study irrelevant to the United States.

Along this same line, James Rachels has argued that our society allows killing in self-defense, and this provision has not led to a breakdown in respect for life. If we can distinguish the innocent from the noninnocent in cases of self-defense, why can we not distinguish the voluntary from the nonvoluntary?[15]

Third, the mere fact that abuses are possible does not show that a practice should not be legalized. Some can abuse the self-defense exception; a cold-blooded murderer can make it *appear* that he killed in self-defense. But the crucial issue is whether the evil of abuses would be so great as to outweigh the benefits of the practice in question. The wedge argument is probably the most important objection against the legalization of voluntary euthanasia. But to assess its adequacy, further discussion is needed.

Here we have not tried to resolve the issue of whether voluntary euthanasia should be legalized. But we have reviewed the major objections to it and have noted the responses to these objections. This is a very important issue of public policy that requires further debate.

MORAL ISSUES

Putting aside questions of legalization, is it morally permissible for competent persons to consent to their own deaths?

Suicide and Euthanasia

Let us begin by asking whether voluntary euthanasia and suicide are morally different. The two do have something in common: each is an instance of a person wishing for and seeking death. There is an important difference, however. Suicide directly involves only one party, namely, the person who wants to die; voluntary euthanasia involves a second party, the person who, through an act or omission, hastens the death of the one who wants to die. This difference may be morally relevant since allowing a second party to be the instrument of a person's death opens the door to possible abuses of the sort to which the wedge argument calls attention. This point suggests that some will want to deny the claim that even if suicide is sometimes permissible, then voluntary euthanasia must be permissible too.

On the other hand, it seems quite plausible to say that if suicide is always wrong, then voluntary euthanasia is also always wrong. Suicide is not more morally problematic than voluntary euthanasia, and it may be less problematic. Suppose that suicide is always wrong. What could possibly allow someone else to end your life at your request when you yourself are not permitted to take such an action? This lays the groundwork for an important objection to voluntary euthanasia. Opponents can argue that voluntary euthanasia is impermissible because suicide is always wrong. If they can convince us that suicide is always wrong, they have a forceful objection. To address this objection adequately, defenders of voluntary euthanasia need to do two things. First, they must consider the reasons that critics give to show that suicide is always wrong and demonstrate that those reasons are inadequate. Second, they need to present a positive case to convince us that suicide is at least sometimes permissible.

Many different reasons have been given to support the claim that suicide is always wrong. Some of these are religious in nature and will not be described here. Instead, we will consider two secular arguments designed to show that suicide is impermissible.

The first is called the *natural law argument*. According to this argument, suicide is wrong because it involves a breach of the natural law of self-preservation. This law assumes that doing what is unnatural is wrong. To say that self-preservation is a natural law is to say that each living creature is endowed with the instinct for self-preservation. Yet this argument is difficult to understand. It appears to derive what people ought to do from premises that state what is the case. Some say that all such arguments fail because they commit the naturalistic fallacy, improperly deriving value judgments from factual ones.[16] In any case, this argument rests on a theory of natural law that is highly controversial.

Another approach to this argument is to ask in what sense is the law of self-preservation a law. At least two senses of "law" might be meant here; but, on either account, the natural law argument seems inadequate. The term *natural law* might be used in a descriptive sense. This means that laws describe how things are. Such laws are universal in scope. Newton's laws of gravity are natural laws in this descriptive sense. If the claim that the law of self-preservation is law in the descriptive sense, it is false. Not every being seeks to preserve itself, including those who attempt to commit suicide. Perhaps, then, the term *natural law* is used in a prescriptive sense, which means that the law tells us not how things are but how they ought to be. The law prohibiting the killing of innocent persons is prescriptive. If advocates of the natural law argument intend the law of self-preservation to be understood as prescriptive, then it will not be subject to the simple counterexample described earlier.

It will be open to another objection, however. If the law of self-preservation is taken to be prescriptive, the argument will be question begging. To say that an argument is question begging is to say that it presupposes the truth of the proposition to be proved. If the law of self-preservation is understood to be prescriptive, then it tells us that there is an obligation to preserve oneself. But to say that individuals ought to preserve themselves is just to say that attempting suicide is wrong, which assumes the truth of the conclusion to be established. Thus, the defender of the natural law argument is faced with a dilemma. If the law of self-preservation is said to be descriptive, it appears to be false; and if it is said to be prescriptive, the argument begs the question. Either way, the argument fails.

Let us consider another argument designed to show that suicide is wrong. Some arguments against suicide claim that there is a duty to oneself not to take one's own life. The notion of a duty to oneself, however, is controversial, and some doubt that such a thing exists. The second argument to be considered here, though, tries to show that individuals have duties to others not to commit suicide. This argument appeals to the harm principle. It says that those who commit suicide are harming others and so their acts are wrong. How do those who commit suicide harm others? If they have dependents, those individuals' well-being will be jeopardized. In addition, self-inflicted death may cause family members to be unhappy and shameful. A person's suicide might also deprive others of services the person might have rendered or owed them. It seems plausible to restrict a person's action if it threatens to harm others. So, if committing suicide will harm others, there are grounds for saying that it is wrong.

Recall that proponents of this general line of argument against voluntary euthanasia must show that suicide is always wrong. It is doubtful that this second argument accomplishes that. In some cases, a person's committing suicide will not harm others. The self-inflicted death of the proverbial hermit will deprive no other people of services and will cause no one else to be unhappy. In addition, family members may not be unhappy when one of their own commits suicide—sometimes for admirable reasons, sometimes for dubious reasons.

Moreover, this argument may play fast and loose with the concept of harm. When a person commits suicide, does that person *harm* those family members who feel hurt or ashamed? It is not obvious that every case in which people say correctly that they are adversely affected by an act is also a case in which they are harmed. Suppose that your neighbor is a member of a conservative religious cult. Members of this cult believe that consuming alcoholic beverages is a sin. Your neighbor becomes extremely upset whenever he sees someone else drinking alcoholic beverages. If you sit on your porch and drink beer, are you harming your neighbor simply because he becomes upset? It seems not. Similarly, you are not harming your parents if they become upset because you marry a person of a different race or because you refuse to have your newborn child baptized. The concept of harm is difficult to explain, but the mere fact that an action upsets others is not sufficient to establish that it harms them.

Arguably, the shame or unhappiness that friends and family members experience because of a suicide is also not always properly categorized as harm. To be sure, in *some* cases a suicide does harm others. If a person uses explosives to commit suicide and in so doing injures others, that person violates the harm principle. And if a parent leaves children as survivors who will not be cared for adequately, she too has violated the harm principle. But the point is that once we reflect on the concept of harm, we can see that not all suicides harm others even when others are understandably upset. As a result, the second argument does not show that suicide is always wrong.

The proponents of voluntary euthanasia, then, can plausibly claim that the arguments considered here to show that suicide is always wrong fail. But can any positive reasons be given to convince us that suicide is sometimes permissible? The usual strategy is to appeal to examples. Consider the familiar story of Captain Oates, a member of Robert Scott's expedition to the South Pole. As he and several of his companions were returning from a mission of exploration, Oates had a serious accident and was disabled. The group was far from the depot, their only source of food and shelter. It appeared that if the others continued to help Oates, none would make it back alive. However, if Oates were to detach himself from the group, an act that would ensure a quick death for him, the others would have a good chance to return safely. It seemed that Oates was permitted to do what would result in his quick death. He believed that no matter what he did, he would die relatively soon. If he detached himself from the group, that action, in effect, was suicide. But if he remained with the group, he would hinder their progress, and they would all probably perish. Since Oates was likely to die soon no matter what he did, and since he could save several lives by sacrificing his own, surely he was at least permitted to detach himself from the group. Some might even argue that he is morally required to commit suicide. This stronger claim is controversial, however, because many will say that sacrificial acts are supererogatory, that is, above and beyond the call of duty. But whether the act is obligatory or supererogatory, it surely is at least permissible.

Consider a second case. The plane of a military pilot goes out of control over a heavily populated area. The pilot can either bail out and let the plane fall, thereby endangering the lives of many civilians, or can crashland in an area where no one else will be hurt but ensuring his own death. Surely the latter choice is at least permissible.

These two cases show that sacrificing one's own life for the good of others is sometimes justified. But some have wondered whether these are really cases of committing suicide. Perhaps it is simple-minded to equate sacrificing one's own life with committing suicide.[17] Even if this is so, paradigmatic cases of suicide are justified. Consider the case of a spy or prisoner of war who has been captured by the enemy. This person knows important secrets about our military operations, and if the enemy obtains this information, many innocent lives will be endangered. This person knows that he will be tortured and forced to reveal the information. So, to protect the lives of those innocent persons, he takes a cyanide tablet and dies. This act is suicide, and most will agree that the spy is justified in committing it.

This discussion shows that the objection that voluntary euthanasia is always wrong because suicide is always wrong is not convincing. Not only are the arguments to show that suicide is always wrong not persuasive, but there are positive reasons to believe that suicide is at least sometimes permissible. But this point does not show that voluntary euthanasia is permissible; it merely refutes an objection. And because voluntary euthanasia involves a second party bringing about a person's death while suicide only involves the victim, additional objections to euthanasia may be raised. This consideration suggests that if possible, it is morally preferable to allow a patient to commit suicide rather than to engage in mercy killing. If society takes this option, however, it should be a program of supervised suicide; for it is much more difficult to commit suicide quickly, painlessly, and successfully than many have appreciated.[18]

Codes of Ethics

Suppose that a patient, because of physical weakness or paralysis, is unable to commit suicide. Is euthanasia on request permitted in this case? If a second party is involved in hastening a patient's death, that second party will likely be a health care practitioner. And precisely because of the role that nurses and physicians must play, some have objected to the practice of voluntary euthanasia. Critics argue that physicians and nurses are required to preserve their patients' lives. In particular, they claim that the codes of ethics to which these medical professionals are committed forbid active euthanasia. The Hippocratic Oath, for example, says, "I will neither give a deadly drug to anybody if asked for it, nor will I make a suggestion to this effect." And the International Code of Nursing Ethics states that a nurse's fundamental responsibility is to conserve life. So, the critic concludes, medical professionals are forbidden to assist patients in an act of mercy killing.

This objection, though common, is not convincing. Professional codes of ethics are of necessity oversimplified. It is true that the Hippocratic Oath directs physicians not to participate in euthanasia.[19] But doctors are also required by the oath to benefit the sick to the best of their ability. What is a physician to do if she judges that the best way to benefit a patient with excruciating throat cancer is to end that patient's life on request?

It is also true that the first clause of the International Code of Nursing Ethics states that the nurse is to conserve life. But there is more to the clause. In its entirety, it says, "The fundamental responsibility of the nurse is threefold: to conserve life, to alleviate suffering, and to promote health." Obviously, the obligation to conserve life can conflict with the obligation to alleviate suffering in certain situations. In some cases, the only way to ease a patient's suffering may be to administer a drug so powerful that it will be lethal. What is a nurse required to do when such a conflict arises?

Professional codes of ethics are important and sometimes useful. But their value is limited. They serve as guidelines, but authors of such codes cannot anticipate every kind of situation that might arise for the professional in question. And frequently circumstances arise in which parts of the code will conflict. It is not convincing, therefore, if critics of voluntary euthanasia rest their entire case on the fact that such an activity is proscribed by various codes of ethics. If the same code directs health care professionals to relieve suffering, a conflict will emerge, the resolution of which is not always obvious. We should admit that proponents of these codes may have an additional point in mind—namely, that one means of relieving suffering, killing, may never be employed. If this is the contention, however, then some explanation of its basis is needed.

Patients' Rights

Many other objections are raised against voluntary euthanasia; not all can be considered here. But even if all objections could be reviewed, that is not enough. Positive reasons are needed too. So, we shall conclude this section with an argument designed to show that voluntary euthanasia is sometimes permissible.

This argument is predicated on the assumptions that each person has the rights to life and autonomy and that those rights in turn give people the right to choose whether to continue to live or to die. The argument may be stated as follows:

1. **To possess a right is to possess something that puts a legitimate restraint on the actions of others.**
2. **Because each person has the rights to life and autonomy, each person has the right to choose whether to continue to live or to die, provided that such choice does not interfere with the rights of others.**
3. **So, others may not interfere when a person chooses to die, provided that this choice does not interfere with the rights of others.**

Premise 1 of this argument is a partial analysis of what it means for a person to have a right. Premise 2 states the assumption concerning the rights to life and autonomy. And line 3, which is supported by premises 1 and 2, says that it is wrong not to let a person die if that person has freely chosen to do so. In medical contexts, this observation means that others must honor a person's choice to refuse or discontinue life-sustaining treatment. This applies to voluntary passive euthanasia. If a person has asked that his life not be saved, it is wrong to interfere. Notice that this is simply a case of a competent patient refusing lifesaving therapy, and, as we saw in Chapter 3, good reasons exist for saying that persons have this right.

This argument can be extended in a more controversial direction, however, if the following premise is accepted:

4. **Others may assist a person in exercising his rights if they are asked to do so and they choose to comply.**

With this additional premise, one can derive another conclusion:

5. **So, others may assist a person in exercising his right to carry out the choice to die if they are asked to do so.**

Premise 4 says that a person who has a right is permitted to enlist the aid of others in exercising that right. Line 5, which follows from premises 2 and 4, says, in effect, that voluntary *active* euthanasia is morally *permissible*. If someone asks you to help him exercise the right to die by providing a lethal drug, you are permitted to do so.

One implication of this argument is that in the same situation, passive euthanasia and active euthanasia can have different moral statuses. If a competent patient asks you not to provide life-extending treatment, you are *required* to comply with that person's wishes; but providing positive assistance in hastening that person's death is merely permissible, not required, unless some exceptional circumstance obtains.

This argument—in particular, premise 2—seems to imply that suicide is only wrong if it interferes with the rights of others, and many will find that aspect objectionable. Note, however, that even if suicide is permissible in certain circumstances, it may not be rational. An act that does not violate others' rights may still be irrational and inadvisable. And this argument implies that interference with the person's act is wrong only if that person is competent.

Some hold that euthanasia is wrong because matters of life and death are "God's work"; anyone who practices euthanasia is said to be "playing God."[20] While this perspective cannot be discussed here at length, two points should be noted. First, it is hard to see how *others* are playing God if only voluntary euthanasia is practiced, for voluntary euthanasia lets people call their own shots. Of course, proponents of this objection may say that voluntary euthanasia involves individuals playing God with their own lives. But this view leads to the second point. If matters of life and death are God's work, then saving lives will also constitute an interference. Using elaborate lifesaving machinery certainly seems to be interfering with nature. Yet few oppose these activities.

A more serious objection to this argument concerns its understanding of the rights to life and autonomy. By combining the two, it says that people have not only the right to life but also a right to choose death as long as that interferes with no one else's rights. This opinion is controversial. Perhaps some different understanding of the rights to life and autonomy are more plausible. The argument also seems to portray the right

EUTHANASIA $\parallel$ 133

to life as alienable. For premises 2 and 4 together seem to suggest that a person's consent alone justifies another in taking his life. These premises could be altered, however, so that the possessor's consent was necessary but not alone sufficient to justify hastening death; other requirements could be stipulated, such as the presence of a terminal illness, without destroying the argument's main thrust.

Finally, premise 4 is needed before any conclusion about voluntary *active* euthanasia can be reached, and its truth may be questioned. This premise says that people may enlist the help of others in exercising their rights, which is certainly true in some cases. My property rights may permit me to remove the large tree from my backyard, and I may enlist your assistance in doing so. But this point does not seem to be true of all rights. In virtue of being married, husbands and wives may have certain rights. It does not follow, however, that spouses may have others help them exercise those rights. So further investigation of premise 4 is needed to determine whether it holds of the rights to life and autonomy as proponents of this argument think.

Physician-Assisted Suicide

Physician-assisted suicide occurs when a physician provides a patient with the means and knowledge to commit suicide. For example, the physician may provide the patient with a prescription for barbiturates and knowledge of what constitutes a fatal overdose. By contrast, with voluntary euthanasia the physician not only makes the means available but is also the *agent* of death on the patient's request. In the early 1990s, the activities of Dr. Jack Kevorkian brought the issue of physician-assisted suicide before the public for debate.

We might begin by asking what can be said in defense of the claim that physician-assisted suicide should be permitted. In appropriate circumstances, the practice seems to be supported by two fundamental moral principles. If the patient making the request is competent, then the principle of autonomy suggests that the physician is permitted to help the patient. And if the patient is suffering or if the patient fears the indignities and dependence associated with her terminal illness, then the principle of beneficence seems to support physician-assisted suicide. When one adds that suicide attempts are often unsuccessful and that such patients frequently compound their problems, the case for assistance based on beneficence is even stronger.[21]

Most in the medical establishment oppose physician-assisted suicide. Reasons for this opposition were recently articulated by the American Medical Association's Council on Ethical and Judicial Affairs.[22] Four points stand out in this report. First, the council argues that physician-assisted suicide is an inappropriate extension of the right to refuse treatment. The right to self-determination gives patients the right to accept or refuse offered interventions, but not the right to demand that physicians hasten their deaths. Second, when physicians are dealing with dying patients, they should offer comfort measures and provide whatever pain medications are necessary to control suffering. Third, assisted suicide would involve physicians in making inappropriate value judgments about the quality of life. The physician's role, instead, is to affirm life. Finally, the council invokes the wedge (or slippery slope) argument. They claim that permitting assisted suicide opens the door to policies that carry far too many risks. They say that it will be too easy to move from assisted suicide to euthanasia, and from voluntary euthanasia to nonvoluntary and perhaps even involuntary euthanasia.

Defenders of physician-assisted suicide may find it easy to answer the first three points made by the council. All will agree that the right to refuse treatment does not give patients the right to *require* that physicians assist them in suicide. But the issue is whether physicians are *permitted* to provide such assistance, not whether they are required to do so. All can also agree that whenever possible, comfort care and relief from suffering should be provided. But the problem arises when comfort care is not adequate to deal with the patient's problems. And even the council admits that there are a small number of such cases.

The point that assisted suicide involves physicians in making inappropriate value judgments about the quality of life seems doubtful for two reasons. First, in cases of assisted suicide, the *patient*, not the physician, has decided that his quality of life is such that he no longer wants to live. Second, physicians do have to make judgments about the quality of patients' lives all the time. Consider, for example, when a dying patient is no longer able to make her own decisions. In such a case, the physician must make recommendations to the family, and these recommendations will be based in part on the physician's perception of the patient's quality of life.

Perhaps Dr. Timothy Quill provides the most forceful case in defense of physician-assisted suicide.[23] Quill supports comfort care and approves of assisted suicide only in cases where patients' suffering cannot be adequately controlled or when patients reasonably fear the indignities and dependence likely to be associated with their terminal illness. Quill acknowledges that the wedge argument provides good reason to worry about permitting assisted suicide. But he claims that if strict safeguards are enforced, these worries can be minimized. Thus, Quill approves of assisted suicide only if the following conditions are satisfied:

1. The patient must freely initiate and repeatedly request assistance in death.

2. Psychiatric evaluation must show that the patient's judgment is not distorted.

3. The patient's condition must be incurable and involve intolerable suffering.

4. The patient's suffering must not be the result of inadequate comfort care.

5. Assisted suicide should only occur when the physician has had a standing and meaningful relationship with the patient.

6. Consultation with another physician is required to confirm the patient's diagnosis and prognosis and that the request is voluntary.

7. Documentation to support each of these six conditions is required.

In general, the point of these conditions is to ensure that both autonomy and beneficence support assisted suicide.

Whether Quill has successfully rebutted the wedge argument is arguable. But in concluding this section, it should be noted that Quill joins many others in criticizing Kevorkian's activities. Quill cites these problems.[24] First, Kevorkian is a retired pathologist, not a clinician. So he may not have the knowledge and experience needed to ensure that other medical approaches will not work. Second, he has been willing to act in the absence of a long-standing relationship with the patient. These circumstances suggest that he has not reviewed all of the information about the irreversibility of the patient's illness and about what measures have been tried. Finally, he has assisted patients whose medical conditions have the potential for uncertainty. For example, the highly publicized case of Janet Adkins involved a patient with "early" Alzheimer's disease. So, in assessing the permissibility of physician-assisted suicide, one should keep in mind that not all defenders of the practice approve of the activities of its best-known practitioner.

Recently (1996), two U.S. Circuit Courts, the Ninth and the Second, declared unconstitutional statutes in the states of Washington and New York that absolutely forbid physician-assisted suicide. The Ninth Circuit Court held that competent, terminally ill patients have a liberty-interest in determining the time and manner of their own deaths and that Washington's ban on assisted suicide unconstitutionally restricts the exercise of that liberty. Although physicians should not be prohibited from prescribing medication that will enable terminal patients to end their own lives, the states may *regulate* the activity in order to minimize abuses.

Interestingly, the court mentions favorably many of the safeguards endorsed by Quill. These opinions no doubt will be appealed; we can expect the Supreme Court to address them in 1997.

THE WITHDRAWAL OF LIFESAVING TREATMENT

Not all cases of withdrawing lifesaving treatment are properly described as euthanasia. When we say that an act is one of euthanasia, that seems to imply that alleviation of a patient's pain or suffering prompted the act. But in many cases, life-sustaining treatment is withheld or withdrawn when the patient is not suffering. This occurs most notably in cases where patients are permanently comatose, such as with patients in a persistent vegetative state. Decisions in such cases are a species of a more general problem: making decisions for patients who are not competent. Here we shall restrict ourselves to the cases where others must decide to withhold or withdraw life-sustaining treatment from incompetent patients.

What principles should govern our decisions in these cases?[25] Three basic guidance principles are widely accepted. The first is the *advance directive principle*. It says that in making a decision regarding the treatment, we should do what that patient has explicitly directed while competent. As we saw earlier, patients can accomplish this through living will or medical advance directives. Or patients can determine who will make the decisions by executing a health care power of attorney. This principle extends a competent patient's right of self-determination.

The second principle is the *substituted judgment principle*. It directs surrogate decision makers to choose what the patient would choose if competent and aware of the medical facts and available options. To apply this principle, one must have evidence of what the patient would have wanted. Verbal or written expressions of preferences while competent provide the best evidence. Written evidence would not be in the form of a living will or advance directive, or else the first principle would apply. Instead, it might be a letter to a friend or relative or perhaps a commentary on a well-known case, such as Quinlan. This principle too is based on the patient's right of self-determination.

The third is the *best interest principle*, based on beneficence. It tells us that in making decisions regarding the treatment of incompetents, we should do what is in the best interests of those individuals.

These three principles are lexically ordered: if the first is applicable, it takes priority; if the first is not applicable but the second is, it takes priority; the third is appealed to only when the first two are inapplicable. We should also note that applying the substituted judgment principle requires care. Anecdotal evidence is often introduced to show that a certain patient would (or would not) want a certain treatment. We should be careful to verify that evidence really exists that this is what the *patient* would have wanted; absent such care, we do not promote self-determination.[26] We should also note that determining what course of treatment will best promote a patient's interests is not always obvious. Even when the applicable principle is clear, many decisions will be difficult.

We shall look at cases illustrating these principles. But before doing that, you might wonder how it could ever be in an incompetent patient's best interests to withhold or withdraw life-sustaining treatment. There seem to be several kinds of cases where such a decision does support the patient's best interests. First, if the patient is going to die soon no matter what is done, and if the treatment involves distress—say, because it is invasive—then arguably that treatment is contrary to the patient's best interests, even if it would extend the patient's life briefly. Second, if the burdens of receiving treatment outweigh the benefits, then that treatment is not in the patient's best interests. For example, treatment may extend the patient's life but cause great discomfort; if so, that treatment may not offer a net benefit. Finally, the patient's condition may be such that no treatment can be beneficial. An example is a patient who is in a persistent vegetative state. If this patient will never regain consciousness, then presumably treatment can neither benefit nor harm the patient.

Concerning patients in persistent vegetative states, the following objection might be raised. We can never be certain that such a patient will not regain consciousness. And since the treatment causes no discomfort, it is in the patient's interests to be kept alive. As long as there is any chance, no matter how small, that the prognosis is wrong, then the patient is better off being kept alive as long as she feels no discomfort. This objection, however, overlooks two points.[27] First, to determine what best promotes the patient's interests, we must not only take into account the small probability that she will return to a cognitive state; we must also factor in the high probability that the individual will be severely disabled if she regains consciousness, as the very small number of documented cases fitting here demonstrates. Second, when the probability of returning to a cognitive state is small, society does not have an obligation to keep the patient alive indefinitely. If someone is lost at sea, until the body is recovered there is always a chance that the person is alive. But we do not criticize the family or society for giving up after a reasonable period of time. Here, as in medical cases, great expenditures in the face of overwhelming odds are not morally mandated.

In concluding this chapter, we shall consider three cases to which the aforementioned principles apply. No case will be discussed involving the advance directive principle. If a patient has a living will and/or medical advance directive, and if it is clear how this applies to the patient's case, then the patient's wishes should be followed. In these three cases, none of the patients was dead by the whole-brain concept of death.

The Case of Paul Brophy[28]

Paul Brophy was a firefighter and emergency medical technician who lived in Massachusetts. In March 1983, he suffered a ruptured brain artery. Surgery was performed, but he never regained consciousness. He was transferred to New England Sinai Hospital, and his condition was diagnosed as a persistent vegetative state. Later that year, Brophy's wife gave physicians permission to insert a feeding tube into his stomach. Artificial feeding was continued throughout the next year, with Brophy's condition remaining unchanged.

Early in 1985, Brophy's wife asked physicians to stop the artificial nutrition. She was Catholic and a nurse, and this was a difficult decision for her. But Paul Brophy had often told family members that he did not want to be kept alive if he were permanently comatose. In discussions of the Karen Quinlan case, he had said that he did not want to be sustained that way. And he had had such conversations with his wife, several siblings, and many of his children. The wife's decision to ask that artificial nutrition be stopped was supported by their five children, Brophy's seven siblings, and his elderly mother.

In spite of this unanimity, the physician-in-chief at the hospital would not go along with the request. Mrs. Brophy sought court intervention. This case was typically drawn out, but in September 1986, the Supreme Court of Massachusetts ruled in a split decision (4 to 3) that Paul Brophy's feeding tube could be removed. They did not require the hospital to compromise its principles, however. Instead, they gave the hospital the option of transferring Brophy to another institution. That is what they did, and Paul Brophy died on October 23, 1986.

This case illustrates a clear application of the substituted judgment principle. The evidence suggested that Paul Brophy had expressed his wishes, while competent, many times to many people. At one point, he had even expressed dismay over having saved a man from a burning truck because that man suffered for months before dying. Unless an incredible conspiracy was at work among many people who loved Paul Brophy, the evidence of what he would have wanted is clear. The decision of the Supreme Court of Massachusetts was in accord with the principle of substituted judgment and promoted self-determination.

The Case of Joseph Saikewicz[29]

In 1976, sixty-seven-year-old Joseph Saikewicz was diagnosed as having acute myeloblastic monocytic leukemia. The prognosis was that this illness was incurable and fatal. In approximately 30 to 50 percent of such cases, chemotherapy can bring about remission, but only for two to thirteen months.

Saikewicz had an IQ of approximately ten and had been institutionalized for more than fifty years. His mental age was less than three years. Because of his retardation, he was not able to communicate verbally. His only responses were gestures and grunts. When given medical treatments, he could not respond to questions about whether he was experiencing pain. He became upset when removed from his only familiar environment. His only known family members were two sisters, and they preferred to have no involvement in any decisions concerning him.

A guardian *ad litem* was appointed to determine whether chemotherapy should be initiated. The guardian *ad litem* (that is, for the suit or action) cited a number of factors to support the claim that the burdens of chemotherapy would likely outweigh the benefits for Saikewicz: (1) a low chance of producing remission; (2) the certainty that the treatment would cause suffering and adverse side effects; (3) elderly patients have a more difficult time tolerating chemotherapy; (4) Saikewicz was unable to cooperate with his treatment; and (5) he would be unable to understand why this was being done to him, thereby exacerbating his suffering. This is a plausible application of the best interest principle.

The Supreme Court of Massachusetts ruled that the decision to withhold chemotherapy from Joseph Saikewicz was proper. But, surprisingly, the court attempted to apply the substituted judgment principle; they attempted to determine what Saikewicz would have wanted were he competent. This makes no sense because Joseph Saikewicz was never competent to develop informed preferences. For someone who was never competent, the only applicable principle is best interests.

The Case of Nancy Cruzan

On January 11, 1983, twenty-five-year-old Nancy Cruzan was in an automobile accident. She was thrown from her vehicle face-down in a ditch. By the time paramedics arrived, her brain had been without oxygen for at least twelve minutes, possibly as long as twenty minutes. She was revived at the scene of the accident and taken to a hospital. She was in a vegetative state from the time of the accident until her death.

In early February 1983, a feeding tube was implanted in Cruzan at Freeman Hospital in Joplin, Missouri. Later that month, she was transferred to Brady Rehabilitation Center, and in October 1983 she was taken to Missouri Rehabilitation Center in Mt. Vernon, Missouri.

At the time of her accident, Nancy Cruzan was married. But the marriage was troubled, and in January 1984, Cruzan's parents, Joseph and Joyce Cruzan, were granted guardianship. Later that year they obtained a divorce in their daughter's behalf.

Late in 1984, Cruzan still had not regained consciousness, and the family brought her home for Christmas in the hope that familiar surroundings would produce positive results. They did not.

By the fall of 1986, the family had reached the conclusion that Cruzan would never regain consciousness and that her feeding tube should be removed. But they proceeded slowly. Early in 1987 they sought legal assistance from the American Civil Liberties Union, and in May of that year they contacted William Colby, an attorney who would serve as their lawyer throughout the case. On May 28, 1987, they hand-delivered a formal request to Missouri Rehabilitation Center (MRC) to stop all artificial nutrition and hydration. This action was opposed by MRC, and in March 1988 a hearing was held. On July 27, 1988, the judge ruled in favor of the Cruzans. But the case was appealed, and on November 16, 1988, the Missouri Supreme Court overturned the judge's decision and ruled against the Cruzans. Missouri law did not allow the withdrawal of nutrition or hydration from an incompetent patient unless there was clear and compelling evidence that this is what the patient would have wanted. The Cruzans had testified about their daughter's general outlook on life but did not satisfy the standard of clear and compelling evidence. In July 1989, the U.S. Supreme Court agreed to hear this case. Oral arguments were made on December 6, 1989, and on June 25, 1990, the U.S. Supreme Court upheld the Missouri Supreme Court ruling (in a 5–4 split decision).

In the meantime, two former coworkers of Cruzan had come forward, claiming that in conversations she had indicated that she would not want to be maintained like Karen Quinlan. Various reasons explained why they had not come forward sooner. In one case, the former coworker knew Cruzan under her married name and did not realize that it was she until the case was on appeal. In the other, the person thought that families made these decisions. In any case, this was new evidence, and so the Cruzans renewed their request for a discontinuance of life-sustaining treatment on August 30, 1990. In September, the Missouri Attorney General withdrew from the case, thereby opening the door for the Cruzans. On December 14, 1990, the judge ruled that Cruzan's feeding tubes should be removed in compliance with the family's request. That occurred. Right-to-life protestors stormed MRC on December 18, but the family's wishes prevailed. On December 26, 1990, nearly eight years after the accident, Nancy Cruzan was pronounced dead.

What principles apply here? Since Cruzan had executed no legal documents, the advance directive principle was not relevant. Was substituted judgment the applicable principle? Testimony of family members and coworkers may suggest an affirmative answer to this question, but allowing anecdotal testimony as evidence for what the patient would have wanted if competent is dangerous. Standards for evidence should be high here. In the case of Paul Brophy, there was a variety of sources and the evidence was compelling. In the Cruzan case, that point seems more doubtful. If so, the best interest principle should be employed.

Can that principle, however, justify withdrawing nutrition and hydration from an incompetent patient? It can. A patient in a persistent vegetative state whose wishes are not known arguably is neither benefited nor harmed by medical treatment. In such cases, it seems entirely plausible to allow the family to decide what to do. Indeed, the biggest problem might occur if the family wants the patient sustained indefinitely. Such medical treatment serves no good medical purpose and seems futile. Though society collectively needs to address this issue, it is not obvious that families should have a right to demand such treatment.

Some were very upset when nutrition and hydration were withdrawn from Nancy Cruzan because they believed she would suffer a horrible death. But physicians have long believed that patients in persistent vegetative states experience neither pleasure nor pain. And credence was lent to the claim that Cruzan did not suffer by a recent study published in a prestigious medical journal.[30] Physician Louise Printz argues that withdrawing hydration from patients who are near death does not add to their discomfort. Indeed, withdrawing hydration may even have an analgesic effect because of the accompanying increase of opioids, substances occurring naturally in the body that act on the brain to decrease pain. Printz says that in some situations, physicians can actually help to prevent a slow, painful death by not administering medical hydration.

The best interest principle is the one best applicable to the Cruzan case, and it permits withdrawing life-sustaining treatment, including nutrition and hydration, from a patient in a persistent vegetative state.

WITHHOLDING VERSUS WITHDRAWING TREATMENT

Withdrawing life-sustaining treatment is stopping a medical intervention some time after it has been initiated. Withholding life-sustaining treatment is choosing not to start it. Health care practitioners are often said to find withdrawing treatment to be more difficult to justify than withholding treatment; in withdrawing, they feel that they are killing the patient. But in spite of these common feelings, a growing consensus among ethicists is that withdrawing treatment is *not* ethically worse than withholding treatment, and in some cases there are good reasons for starting treatment and then being willing to withdraw it rather than not starting at all. Among these reasons are the following.[31]

First, starting treatment enables health care professionals to make a fuller, more definitive evaluation of their patients' conditions. To resolve many uncertainties requires time. Second, there is no duty to continue treatment once it has been demonstrated to be ineffective, but sometimes a trial of therapy is needed to determine if treatment will work. Finally, a *policy* that makes withholding treatment easier than withdrawing it may prompt some physicians to withhold treatment too often, and such a policy is contrary to the best interests of patients. For these reasons, withdrawing treatment is typically not regarded as morally worse than withholding that same treatment.

SUMMARY

In discussing euthanasia, we must distinguish between active and passive euthanasia. The received view is that active euthanasia is either always wrong or at least more difficult to justify than passive euthanasia. James Rachels challenges this view, arguing that, in the same circumstances, if passive euthanasia is permissible, then so is active euthanasia.

Distinguishing between voluntary and nonvoluntary euthanasia is also important. Most agree that voluntary euthanasia is easier to justify than nonvoluntary euthanasia, but a problem arises in understanding what is meant by "voluntary euthanasia." Several different accounts of this concept are available, and which we adopt makes a practical difference. The most narrow understanding of voluntary euthanasia better ensures protection against possible abuse but allows for euthanasia in relatively few cases. The broader understanding allows for more instances of euthanasia but is more likely to lead to abuses.

Because euthanasia involves one human being playing a role in the death of another, society must regulate the activity. To evaluate legislation on euthanasia, lawmakers must ask of each proposal who may be euthanized, whether it allows only for voluntary euthanasia, whether it allows only for passive euthanasia, and what safeguards are included. Opponents object to legalizing voluntary euthanasia for many reasons: they say that suffering must be prevented without hastening death, that it is difficult to tell when consent is genuine, that the victim's consent does not justify killing, that judgments about terminal illnesses may be mistaken, and that allowing euthanasia will lead to too many abuses. Defenders of voluntary euthanasia retort that suffering cannot always be prevented without hastening death, that experienced practitioners can usually tell when consent is genuine, that consent in selected cases may justify killing, and that safeguards can minimize the likelihood of diagnostic errors and render improbable the occurrence of abuses.

Against the morality of mercy killing, some argue that since suicide is always wrong, voluntary euthanasia is always wrong too. But this objection is not fully convincing because common arguments to show that suicide is always wrong are weak, and in some cases suicide seems permissible. Because both beneficence and autonomy lend some support to voluntary euthanasia, the burden of proof is on opponents to show why the practice is impermissible.

Finally, withdrawing life-sustaining treatment from unconscious patients is not considered euthanasia because it is not designed to relieve patients' suffering. In making such decisions for incompetent patients, we usually employ three lexically ordered principles: the advance directive principle, the substituted judgment principle, and the best interest principle. The advance directive principle instructs surrogates to act in accord with a patient's living will or health care power of attorney, if such a document exists. The substituted judgment principle directs surrogates to make decisions for incompetents by trying to determine what that patient would have wanted were he competent, assuming that no legally executed directive exists. This principle was properly followed in the case of Paul Brophy, who had independently informed his wife, children, and siblings that he would not want to be maintained in a vegetative state. If no advance directive exists and it is not feasible to determine what the patient would have wanted, then surrogates should make medical decisions based on what is in the patient's best interest. The case of Joseph Saikewicz illustrates the application of this principle.

Suggestions for Further Reading

Battin, Margaret. "Voluntary Euthanasia and the Risks of Abuse: Can We Learn Anything from the Netherlands?" *Law, Medicine, & Health Care*, Vol. 20 (1992), pp. 133–143.

Beauchamp, Tom L. "Suicide." In Tom Regan (ed.), *Matters of Life and Death*, 2d ed. (New York: Random House, 1986), pp. 77–124.

Beauchamp, Tom L., and James F. Childress. *Principles of Biomedical Ethics*, 4th ed. (New York: Oxford University Press, 1994), Chapter 4.

Buchanan, Allen E., and Dan W. Brock. *Deciding for Others: The Ethics of Surrogate Decision Making* (New York: Cambridge University Press, 1989).

Cundiff, David. *Euthanasia Is Not the Answer* (Totowa, NJ: Humana, 1992).

Dworkin, Ronald. *Life's Dominion* (New York: Knopf, 1993).

Feinberg, Joel. "Voluntary Euthanasia and the Inalienable Right to Life." In *Rights, Justice, and the Bounds of Liberty* (Princeton, NJ: Princeton University Press, 1980), pp. 221–251.

Foot, Philippa. "The Problem of Abortion and the Doctrine of Double Effect." In *Virtues and Vices* (Berkeley: University of California Press, 1978), pp. 19–32.

McConnell, Terrance. "The Nature and Basis of Inalienable Rights." *Law and Philosophy*, Vol. 3 (1984), pp. 25–59.

Pence, Gregory E. *Classic Cases in Medical Ethics* (New York: McGraw-Hill, 1990), Chapters 1 and 3.

Quill, Timothy E. *Death and Dignity* (New York: Norton, 1993).

Rachels, James. "Active and Passive Euthanasia." In Ronald Munson (ed.), *Intervention and Reflection: Basic Issues in Medical Ethics*, 4th ed. (Belmont, CA: Wadsworth, 1992), pp. 163–167.

Rachels, James. *The End of Life* (New York: Oxford University Press, 1986).

Rachels, James. "More Impertinent Distinctions and a Defense of Active Euthanasia." In Thomas A. Mappes and Jane S. Zembaty (eds.), *Biomedical Ethics*, 3d ed. (New York: McGraw-Hill, 1991), pp. 374–381.

Steinbock, Bonnie. "The Intentional Termination of Life." In John Arras and Nancy Rhoden (eds.), *Ethical Issues in Modern Medicine*, 3d ed. (Mountain View, CA: Mayfield, 1991), pp. 245–250.

Notes

1. I ignore here two other moral categories of actions, namely, the supererogatory and the offensive. A *supererogatory* action is one that is above and beyond the call of duty; it is morally desirable but not required. An *offensive* act is one that is morally undesirable but not forbidden.

2. James Rachels, "Active and Passive Euthanasia," in Ronald Munson (ed.), *Intervention and Reflection: Basic Issues in Medical Ethics*, 4th ed. (Belmont, CA: Wadsworth, 1992), pp. 163–167.

3. This criticism is by Bonnie Steinbock, "The Intentional Termination of Life," in John Arras and Nancy Rhoden (eds.), *Ethical Issues in Modern Medicine*, 3d ed. (Mountain View, CA: Mayfield, 1989), pp. 245–250.

4. Consensus is growing among bioethicists that the old distinction between ordinary and extraordinary care is not helpful and that the focus should be on whether the treatment provides the patient with more benefits than burdens. See *Guidelines on the Termination of Life-Sustaining Treatment and the Care of the Dying* (Bloomington: Indiana University Press, 1987), p. 5.

5. See *Guidelines on the Termination of Life-Sustaining Treatment and the Care of the Dying*, p. 73.

6. See *Guidelines on the Termination of Life-Sustaining Treatment and the Care of the Dying*, pp. 128–129.

7. James Rachels, "More Impertinent Distinctions and a Defense of Active Euthanasia," in Thomas A. Mappes and Jane S. Zembaty (eds.), *Biomedical Ethics*, 3d ed. (New York: McGraw-Hill, 1991), pp. 374–381.

8. See Philippa Foot, "The Problem of Abortion and the Doctrine of Double Effect," in *Virtues and Vices* (Berkeley: University of California Press, 1978), pp. 19–32.

9. For a discussion of the safeguards employed in the practice of mercy killing in Holland, see Gregory E. Pence, *Classic Cases in Medical Ethics* (New York: McGraw-Hill, 1990), pp. 51–52.

10. See David Cundiff, *Euthanasia Is Not the Answer* (Totowa, NJ: Humana, 1992). Cundiff's argument seems to be aimed against *active* euthanasia.

11. For a detailed discussion of these two versions of the wedge argument, see Tom L. Beauchamp and James F. Childress, *Principles of Biomedical Ethics*, 4th ed. (New York: Oxford University Press, 1994), pp. 229–231.

12. The points in this paragraph in response to the first objection are made forcefully by Timothy E. Quill, *Death and Dignity* (New York: Norton, 1993), especially Chapters 5 and 6.

13. For two different approaches that adopt this strategy, see Joel Feinberg, "Voluntary Euthanasia and the Inalienable Right to Life," in *Rights, Justice, and the Bounds of Liberty* (Princeton, NJ: Princeton University Press, 1980), pp. 221–251; and Terrance McConnell, "The Nature and Basis of Inalienable Rights," *Law and Philosophy*, Vol. 3 (1984), pp. 25–59.

14. See Margaret Battin, "Voluntary Euthanasia and the Risks of Abuse: Can We Learn Anything from the Netherlands?" *Law, Medicine, & Health Care*, Vol. 20 (1992), pp. 133–143.

15. James Rachels, *The End of Life* (New York: Oxford University Press, 1986), pp. 174–175.

16. For a discussion of the naturalistic fallacy, see William K. Frankena, *Ethics*, 2d ed. (Upper Saddle River, NJ: Prentice Hall, 1973), pp. 99–100.

17. For a discussion of these issues, see Tom L. Beauchamp, "Suicide," in Tom Regan (ed.), *Matters of Life and Death*, 2d ed. (New York: Random House, 1986), pp. 77–124.

18. On this point, see Pence, *Classic Cases in Medical Ethics*, pp. 36–37.

19. The historical origins of the Hippocratic Oath are curious, and the evidence suggests that many of its components were not endorsed by the majority of practicing physicians in ancient Greece. For an illuminating discussion, see Ludwig Edelstein, *The Hippocratic Oath: Text, Translation, and Interpretation* (Baltimore: Johns Hopkins University Press, 1943).

20. I consider this point here as it is usually presented in "popular" contexts. Within the context of theological ethics, the matter is far more complex. For a helpful discussion, see Robert Wennberg, *Terminal Choices* (Grand Rapids, MI: Eerdmans, 1989). Another, perhaps more charitable, interpretation of this objection is that its proponents are asserting that human life is sacred. For a detailed discussion of this doctrine, see Ronald Dworkin, *Life's Dominion* (New York: Knopf, 1993), Chapter 3.

21. See Quill, *Death and Dignity*, pp. 116, 134–135.

22. AMA Council on Ethical and Judicial Affairs, *Code of Medical Ethics Reports*, July 1994, pp. 269–275.

23. Points in this paragraph are taken from Quill, *Death and Dignity*, Chapter 8, especially pp. 161–165.

24. Quill, *Death and Dignity*, pp. 124–125.

25. The discussion here draws from what is by far the definitive work on this topic: Allen E. Buchanan and Dan W. Brock, *Deciding for Others* (New York: Cambridge University Press, 1989), especially pp. 93–134.

26. Recent studies raise doubts about the accuracy of substituted judgment. For one example, see Allison Seckler, Diane Meier, Michael Mulvihill, and Barbara Paris, "Substituted Judgment: How Accurate Are Proxy Predictions?" *Annals of Internal Medicine*, Vol. 115 (1991), pp. 92–97.

27. This response is made in Buchanan and Brock, *Deciding for Others*, pp. 130–132.

28. *Brophy v. New England Sinai Hospital, Inc.*, 497 N.E. 2d 626 (Massachusetts 1986). For a discussion of this case, see Beauchamp and Childress, *Principles of Biomedical Ethics*, pp. 522–524, and Buchanan and Brock, *Deciding for Others*, pp. 126–127.

29. *Superintendent of Belchertown v. Saikewicz*, 370 N.E. 2d 417 (Massachusetts 1977). For a discussion of this case, see Beauchamp and Childress, *Principles of Biomedical Ethics*, p. 522, and Buchanan and Brock, *Deciding for Others*, pp. 113–115, 124–126.

30. Louise Printz, "Terminal Hydration, a Compassionate Treatment," *Archives of Internal Medicine*, Vol. 152 (1992), pp. 697–700.

31. See Terrance McConnell and Rita Layson, "Buying Time," in Kenneth Iserson, Arthur Sanders, and Deborah Mathieu (eds.), *Ethics in Emergency Medicine*, 2d ed. (Tucson, AZ: Galen, 1995), pp. 197–203.

CHAPTER 5

Abortion

WHEN THE HUMAN FEMALE reproductive cell, the *ovum*, is fertilized by the male sex cell, the *spermatozoon*, the product is called the *zygote*, a single-celled being containing forty-six chromosomes. Within the first days of conception, the zygote begins to divide. By the third day, it normally consists of sixteen cells. As the zygote begins to grow during the first week, it moves through the Fallopian tube into the uterus. If the zygote fails to descend into the uterus and continues to develop in the Fallopian tube, pregnancy is called *ectopic* and normally must be terminated. At this point, as the zygote is gradually implanted in the uterine wall, it is called the *conceptus*. From the second through the eighth weeks of growth, it is called the *embryo*. From the third month until birth, it is called the *fetus*. In ordinary discourse, the term *fetus* is often used to refer to the product of conception at any stage of development. When the fetus is capable of surviving outside the womb, it is said to be *viable*.

When the product of conception is expelled from the uterus prematurely, this is called *abortion*. When expulsion is natural, rather than intentional, it is called *spontaneous abortion*, or more commonly, a *miscarriage*. There are several different methods of performing nonspontaneous, elective abortions. One method is the so-called "morning after" pill. Once a fiction, this drug is now a reality with the recent development in France of RU 486, a drug that prevents the zygote from implanting in the uterine wall. Another method of abortion is *uterine aspiration*, a process in which the cervix is dilated, a small tube is inserted into the uterus, and its contents are emptied by suction. Another common procedure is *dilation and curettage* (D and C), which involves dilating the cervix and using a curette (a surgical instrument) to remove its contents. Yet another method of abortion involves the injection of a saline solution into the sac containing the amniotic fluid that surrounds the fetus, which induces a miscarriage. Because elective abortion normally ends the life of a being that is biologically human (that is, it has the same genetic code as any normal member of the species *Homo sapiens*), many questions have been raised about the permissibility of such a procedure.

THE MORAL ISSUES

At what point of fetal development, if any, and for what reasons, if any, is abortion morally permissible?[1] Putting the question this way conveys that two basic issues lie at the heart of the debate about abortion. The first of these issues concerns the stage of fetal development. Many hold that this is a relevant factor in determining the permissibility of abortion and that later abortions are more problematic morally than earlier abortions. The second basic issue concerns the reason that a woman might have for seeking an abortion. To many, some reasons seem more acceptable than others.

Why do people disagree so vehemently about abortion? Opponents in the abortion debate typically disagree about the moral status of the fetus. They disagree about whether fetuses have any rights and, if so, when they acquire those rights. Conservatives hold that fetuses have the full complement of moral rights, including the right to life, from the moment of conception. There is, therefore, a presumption that killing fetuses is wrong. By contrast, liberals claim that fetuses lack moral status. This position maintains that fetuses have none of the rights that adult human beings possess. The fetus is a piece of tissue in the woman's body, and so removing it is no more objectionable morally than removing the appendix. Moderates hold a position between these two extremes. Some moderates claim that in early stages of development fetuses do not possess moral rights, but in later stages they do. According to this position, at some point in their continuous development fetuses acquire moral rights. The moral status of fetuses, then, is one of the major sources of controversy in the debate about abortion.

Even among those who agree that abortion is sometimes permissible, disagreement persists about what reasons justify abortion. Here we shall discuss some of the common reasons that have been advanced to justify abortions.

One set of reasons offered to justify some abortions are called *therapeutic*.[2] Therapeutic abortions are performed for medical reasons. Abortions performed to save the life of the woman or preserve her physical or mental health are therapeutic. Therapeutic abortions are the least controversial.

A second set of reasons to justify abortion are *eugenic*. These reasons are invoked when pregnancy will produce a severely deformed child. Here one might appeal to the interests of both the parents and the fetus to justify abortion. To the extent that it is plausible to appeal to the interests of the fetus itself to justify eugenic abortions, we might describe the act as "fetal euthanasia." People might disagree about when an abortion is properly described as "eugenic." Possible conditions for invoking this reason include Tay-Sachs disease, sickle-cell anemia, and anencephaly.

A third set of reasons to justify some abortions are *humanitarian*. They apply when pregnancy is the result of incest or rape. Many will assimilate these reasons with therapeutic ones; they will point out that fetuses that are the product of an incestuous relation are more likely to have genetic deformities and that if women who have been impregnated due to rape are compelled to carry the fetus to term, their emotional distress is more likely to be exacerbated. But this rationale constitutes a third set of reasons because these connections are not necessary. Pregnancy due to incest does not necessarily produce a deformed child. And many say that *even if* a woman did not experience additional trauma by carrying to term a fetus resulting from rape, considerations of fairness alone suggest that she should be permitted to have an abortion because the pregnancy was involuntary.

A fourth set of reasons to justify some abortions are *socioeconomic*. This category includes permitting an abortion because a woman already has many children, or because she and her family are poor and cannot afford to care for the child, or because the child is unwanted and will therefore likely be unhappy. Reasons that fall in the socioeconomic category are most easily defended from a utilitarian perspective. These are typically situations where no matter what is done, some bad consequences will ensue. To the extent that we might plausibly say that abortion is permissible in these cases, we may do so because it is the least evil of the alternatives.

Though these four reasons are broad and can encompass many subcategories, they do not necessarily exhaust the field. Another reason for having abortions is relatively new.[3] *Amniocentesis* is the process of withdrawing and analyzing amniotic fluid surrounding the fetus. It is normally used to detect genetic defects; however, it also reveals the gender of the fetus. Some couples have used amniocentesis to determine the fetus's gender and have chosen abortion when the fetus is not of the preferred gender. Whether a moral justification exists for this practice is doubtful.

Each of these reasons will justify abortions only in certain situations; that is, even if these reasons are accepted, abortion will be justified only when certain conditions obtain. Some, however, support a legal policy that extends to women the *legal* right to choose abortion whenever they wish, regardless of its morality. Their underlying assumption is this: People have a legal right to do with their bodies whatever they wish, so a woman may have an abortion for any reason; even if others doubt the *moral* appropriateness of the choice, they have no right to interfere. This stand effectively gives a woman a blank check on the question of abortion. If this justification is adequate for legalizing abortion, other reasons become superfluous, though the moral question remains.

ABORTION AND THE LAW

In January 1973, the United States Supreme Court ruled on the question of abortion.[4] Their ruling declared the restrictive abortion laws of Texas and Georgia unconstitutional and placed restrictions on all states. The Texas case, *Roe v. Wade*, concerned a law that permitted abortion only when it was necessary to save the woman's life. The Georgia case, *Doe v. Bolton*, addressed a statute that allowed abortions only when necessary to protect the woman's health, to prevent the birth of a deformed child, or when pregnancy had resulted from rape. Each of these laws limited the rights of women to have abortions; the Texas law was clearly the more restrictive. Using the fictitious name of Jane Roe, a pregnant single woman challenged the constitutionality of the Texas statute. The pseudonym Jane Doe was used by the woman challenging the Georgia law. In declaring these laws unconstitutional and in stating its position on the issue of abortion, the Court invoked three notions: the woman's right to privacy, the health of the woman, and the potential life of the fetus. Here we shall explain the role of each of these concepts in the 1973 decision.

The Court ruled that the Texas and Georgia statutes violated a woman's right to privacy, a right guaranteed by the Fourteenth Amendment. The right to privacy, the Court argued, is broad enough to encompass a woman's decision whether to terminate her pregnancy. Why did the Court appeal to the right to privacy? It ruled that a woman has the right to do what she wishes as long as other persons are not involved. Because of this right to privacy, it is a woman's decision whether to continue or terminate a pregnancy. Such reasoning is predicated on the assumption that the fetus is not a person; apparently the Court regards the fetus as a part of the woman's body. In fact, Justice Harry Blackmun, author of the majority opinion in *Roe v. Wade*, indicates that if the fetus were a person, then its right to life would be guaranteed by the Fourteenth Amendment and abortion would have to be declared illegal.

Why does the Court assume that the fetus is not a person? The majority opinion contains two comments about the personhood of the fetus. First, Justice Blackmun suggests that because experts in the fields of medicine, philosophy, and theology do not agree on the question of when a being becomes a person (or, as Blackmun puts it, when *life* begins), the judiciary cannot be expected to settle the matter. This comment reveals a skepticism about the prospects of determining when personhood begins. The second comment concerns how the fetus has been regarded by the law in the past. It is claimed that no cases can be cited (as of 1973) in which the fetus has been regarded as a person within the meaning of the Fourteenth Amendment. For example, a fetus has no property rights and must be born alive before it can inherit. Put another way, "the unborn have never been recognized in the law as persons in the whole sense." The upshot of these two comments is this. A consensus prevails in society that women are persons with rights, but no such consensus exists about fetuses. So society should give priority to the wishes of women in cases of conflict.

This case was not the first occasion on which the Supreme Court cited the right to privacy as having relevance to decisions about reproduction. In 1965 the Court ruled in the case of *Griswold v. Connecticut*. The Connecticut statute whose constitutionality was challenged read as follows:

> Any person who uses any drug, medicinal article or instrument for the purpose of preventing conception shall be fined not less than fifty dollars or imprisoned not less than sixty days nor more than one year or be both fined and imprisoned.
>
> Any person who assists, abets, counsels, causes, hires or commands another to commit any offense may be prosecuted and punished as if he were the principal offender.

The Court declared that this statute violated the right to privacy of married couples and declared it unconstitutional.

Though the Court did appeal to a woman's right to privacy to strike down the restrictive abortion laws of Texas and Georgia, it did not go so far to say that *any* restriction on abortion is unconstitutional; that is, the Court did not rule that abortion must be granted on demand. According to the Court, the woman's right to privacy is not the only relevant consideration. The state also has a legitimate interest in protecting women's health. During the first trimester of pregnancy, however, the state may not interfere at all with a woman's decision to have an abortion. A medical reason was given to bolster this judgment: The mortality rate for women having an abortion during the first trimester is lower than mortality in normal childbirth.

A state may, however, enact legislation to protect the woman's health during and after the second trimester of pregnancy. As Justice Blackmun puts it, "It follows that, from and after this point [the end of the first trimester], a State may regulate the abortion procedure to the extent that the regulation reasonably relates to the preservation and protection of maternal health." Blackmun then provides examples of permissible regulation:

> Examples of permissible state regulation in this area are requirements as to the qualifications of the person who is to perform the abortion; as to the licensure of that person; as to the facility in which the procedure is to be performed, that is, whether it must be a hospital or may be a clinic or some other place of less-than-hospital status; as to the licensing of the facility; and the like.

Put another way, because abortion is more dangerous to women during the later stages of pregnancy, states may regulate abortion at this point, but only if those regulations are designed to protect women's health. Such restrictions seem to be paternalistic.

According to Blackmun, there is one other relevant factor in determining what sort of restrictions on abortions states may enforce. The state has a legitimate interest in protecting "the potentiality of human life." Concerning this state interest in potential life, Blackmun argues that the compelling point is at viability—that is, when the fetus is capable of living outside the woman's womb. Viability usually occurs at the beginning of the third trimester, or around the twenty-eighth week of pregnancy. Since, according to the Court, the state has an interest in protecting fetal life after viability, it may forbid abortions during the third trimester. Blackmun puts it this way: "If the State is interested in protecting fetal life after viability, it may go so far as to proscribe abortion during that period except when it is necessary to preserve the life or health of the mother."

One point concerning this aspect of the Court's decision should be noted here. In spite of the Court's earlier claim to be unable to say when life or personhood begins, it appears that the Court has committed itself to the view that there is something magical about viability. The Court does not say this explicitly. Instead, it talks about "potential" life. But such talk is surely a confusion. By any ordinary use of that term, the single-cell zygote is just as much a potential person as a viable fetus. It is tempting to say that for all practical purposes the Court has drawn the line for personhood at viability. Such a claim is not accurate, however. If the Court had actually declared that the fetus is a person at viability, then it would have been compelled to say that its right to life is protected by the Fourteenth Amendment. And this claim, in turn, would require all states to prohibit abortion during the third trimester and treat it as homicide. What the Court actually says, however, is that states are *permitted* to proscribe abortion during the third trimester of pregnancy. Therefore, although the Court is committed to saying that viability is important, it does not say that it is the criterion of personhood.

Let us summarize briefly. The 1973 decision of the Supreme Court says that no state may enact legislation limiting a woman's right to have an abortion during the first trimester of pregnancy. During the second trimester, the only regulations that may be placed on abortion are those designed to ensure the safety of the procedure. In other words, a woman's right to privacy gives her a right to have an abortion during the second trimester of pregnancy, but the state may regulate the procedure to protect the woman's health. Restrictive laws are permitted during the third trimester except in those rare cases where abortion is necessary to protect the woman's life or health. Such restrictions are justified, the Court ruled, because the state has a legitimate interest in protecting "potential life."

ABORTION: THE MORAL POSITIONS

We shall now examine the conservative, liberal, and moderate positions on abortion in more detail. These are positions about the morality of abortion, not its legality. Using these terms may be somewhat misleading because they have connotations broader than intended here, but they are the ones commonly used. Put simply, the conservative position is that abortion is always wrong, or at least it is always wrong unless it is necessary to save the woman's life. According to the liberal position, abortion is permissible at any stage of fetal development and for any reason. Moderates maintain positions between these two extremes.

A warning is in order here. Although we shall be talking about the conservative, liberal, and moderate positions, these labels are misnomers. There are no such things as *the* conservative position, *the* liberal position, and *the* moderate position. Each of these views has been defended by many different and sometimes incompatible arguments. Well-known and interesting arguments for each of the positions have been selected. Only for stylistic simplicity has the word *the* been used to describe these views.

In describing these different views on abortion, some people have employed the following convention. The term *human being* is used to refer to any being with a human genetic code. Thus, any creature conceived by human parents is, at the moment of its conception, a human being. The term *human being* is biological, and as it is used here, no moral conclusions follow directly from the fact that a being is a member of that species. The debate about abortion, properly understood, is not about species membership. If it were, the debate would be silly. So, too, the debate is not about when life begins. The argument concerns when a being has moral standing. Beings with moral standing have rights that others must respect.

The term *person* is used here to describe a being with the full complement of moral rights, the rights that we believe all normal adult human beings possess. *Person* is thus being used in a moral sense; it designates a being with full membership in the moral community, including possession of the right to life. It does not follow automatically that all human beings are persons. Whether fetuses are persons is one of the questions at issue in the debate about abortion. And perhaps some persons are not human, depending on what characteristics are needed to qualify as a person. What is involved here is sometimes called "the line drawing problem." In the continuous development of human beings, where is the moral line, the point at which they come to possess the right to life? (We should note, however, that not all questions about abortion are questions about rights. Considerations of utility may be relevant too.)

Adopting this language of personhood begs no questions on the issue of abortion. Indeed, it should clarify the issues to be discussed. Much ink has been spilled debating when fetuses become human or when life begins. These are biological questions, not moral ones. Some of the key moral issues concern what rights fetuses have and when they acquire those rights. The positions that are discussed here have not uniformly adopted this convention. Where necessary, the language has been altered to conform to the terminology employed here.

The Conservative Position[5]

The most important question in the abortion debate concerns the moral status of the fetus. The conservative deals with this by adopting the following thesis: any being conceived by parents who are persons (that is, beings with the full complement of moral rights) is itself a person from the moment of conception. Because it is assumed that adult human beings are persons, it follows from this thesis that any beings conceived by them are also persons. So, human fetuses are persons. Conservatives believe that if this thesis is established, then abortion at any stage of fetal development is wrong. The argument to show that such a conclusion follows is this:

1. It is (prima facie) wrong to kill persons because they have the right to life.
2. Human fetuses are persons and have the right to life.
3. Therefore, it is wrong to kill human fetuses.
4. To abort human fetuses is normally to kill them.
5. Therefore, it is wrong to abort human fetuses.

This argument appears to be valid; that is, it seems that *if* the premises are true, then the conclusion must be true. Lines 1, 2, and 4 are the premises of this argument. Line 3 follows from lines 1 and 2; line 5 follows from lines 3 and 4. If the *form* of this argument is correct, then what is crucial in evaluating its adequacy is the truth of the three premises. Premise 1 is essentially true by definition, and premise 4 is an empirical claim that is surely correct. The adequacy of this argument, then, depends on the truth of premise 2. The conservative's task is to convince others to adopt the account of personhood that supports premise 2.

How does the conservative try to establish this thesis? One approach is to employ an "eliminative" strategy, which involves considering other criteria of personhood endorsed by opponents and trying to demonstrate that they are inadequate. There is an inherent danger in employing such a strategy. To be convincing, *all* of the competing criteria that might be proposed must be considered. And that anyone can complete such a task is most unlikely, for too many possibilities must be considered. But if conservatives raise serious doubts about the standard accounts of personhood, perhaps they will at least render their view plausible. Even this outcome will not establish the position, however; for the inadequacy of the views of one's opponents is not sufficient to establish one's own position.

Surveying the views of conservatives' opponents might begin with a very liberal account, one that marks birth as the point at which personhood, and with it the right to life, begins. According to this view, abortion at any stage of fetal development does not violate a person's right to life, but infanticide does. Conservatives claim that drawing the line at birth is arbitrary; such a position has no moral basis. There do not appear to be any morally significant differences between eight-month-old fetuses and neonates. The only difference is geographic, which is not morally relevant to a being's moral standing. Moreover, if birth is taken to be the point at which personhood is achieved, then the following claim must be endorsed: a prematurely born child whose biological life (that is, its life since conception) is seven months will have rights that an eight-month-old fetus does not have. This claim seems arbitrary and unacceptable, especially given that the fetus is likely more developed. As a result, to say that birth is the point at which human beings acquire rights does not seem plausible.

Let us consider a more moderate criterion. Viability is a popular place to draw the line for when human fetuses acquire the right to life. According to this view, when a fetus is capable of living outside the womb, it is a person and killing it is wrong. As described earlier, the Supreme Court attached a great deal of importance to viability, though it did not ascribe the right to life to viable fetuses. Many who want to say that abortions in later stages of pregnancy are wrong but that early abortions are permissible are inclined to endorse viability as the point at which the right to life begins. What are conservatives' criticisms of this criterion?

First, if artificial incubation is perfected, then fetuses will be viable at any time. In any case, as technology improves, viability will continue to be achieved at an earlier age. This fact is troubling because it suggests that if viability is taken as the criterion of personhood, then a being's moral status depends on the state of technology of that being's society. This point introduces too much relativity into a fundamental moral notion. Proponents of viability may respond that they mean natural viability, but it is not clear what "natural" means here. In any case, other criticisms emerge.

Different fetuses are viable at different ages. This fact holds true, of course, for individual fetuses, but there are also racial differences.[6] Some scientists claim that Negroid fetuses are typically viable several weeks before Caucasian fetuses. If viability is accepted as the criterion of personhood, different beings will acquire moral rights at different times. This sort of variability seems to make viability unworkable as a social policy.

There is a third and related criticism. A previable fetus is absolutely dependent on the woman for its life. But dependence is not ended at viability. Children are dependent on others for years after their births; they cannot survive if others do not tend to their needs. Of course, one difference is evident: a previable fetus is dependent on one particular person for survival, whereas a viable fetus is dependent on someone or other to nurture and care for it. But such a difference seems morally insignificant, and certainly it is not great enough to warrant the claim that a viable fetus has a right to life but a previable fetus does not.

Finally, something is strange about employing viability as the criterion for personhood. Those who adopt this view hold that previable fetuses lack moral rights and so may be aborted, whereas viable fetuses possess rights and may not be aborted. The difference between previable and viable fetuses is that only the former are absolutely dependent on pregnant women for their continued existence. But therein lies the moral oddity. Normally, greater dependence is associated with greater obligations. The obligations of parents toward their children are greater when those children are young and not able to fend for themselves. As the children grow older and more independent, the parents have fewer obligations. The proponent of viability as the criterion for when a being acquires the right to life, though, suggests that no obligations are owed to the fetus as long as it is absolutely dependent on the woman for its life. Because this view reverses moral considerations as we know them in other contexts, some justification is needed. But seldom is one forthcoming. For these reasons, then, conservatives reject the criterion of viability.

Experience or simple consciousness is another criterion for when a being acquires the right to life, one that might support a moderate position. The underlying idea is that beings who are capable of having experiences have special claims. So consciousness is the point at which human beings come to possess the right to life.

Conservatives reject this criterion first by pointing out that it may not serve moderates in the way that they think. Conservatives claim that fetuses have experiences as early as the eighth week after conception. The evidence cited to support this is that fetuses respond to touch at this point of development. Whether this counts as having experience or being conscious is debatable. But if it is taken as such evidence, then the right to life will begin earlier than proponents of this criterion have supposed.

Conservatives' second criticism is more direct. They argue that accepting consciousness as the criterion for when beings acquire the right to life has unacceptable consequences. We will have to say that adult human beings who are permanently comatose or in a persistent vegetative state do not have the right to life. Whether this consequence follows is debatable; for proponents of this criterion might hold that once beings attain consciousness, they have the right to life until they die. Moreover, some will not find counterintuitive the claim that persons permanently comatose or in a persistent vegetative state no longer have the right to life. As a result, these criticisms may not be good ones.

Having supposedly eliminated the competing views, conservatives accept the position that fetuses possess the right to life from the moment of conception. However, the following objection might be raised against this version of the conservative's view. If the single-cell zygote is a person with the right to life, how can we not also say that the sperm and egg have the right to life too? Does not consistency require that conservatives say this? This interpretation is taken as a criticism because it shows that the position leads to absurd results: all forms of birth control are wrong because they deny to the sperm and the egg their right to life.[7]

Some conservatives have tried to show that their position does not lead to this absurd consequence.[8] They want to convince you that drawing the line at conception is not arbitrary; there is a morally relevant difference between zygotes, on the one hand, and sperm and eggs, on the other. To convince you of this, conservatives appeal to probabilities. In the normal male ejaculate, there are as many as 100 to 200 million spermatozoa. In females, at birth ovaries contain a large number of primordial egg cells, anywhere from 100,000 to 1,000,000. A woman ovulates about 13 times per year for approximately 30 years, so only about 390 to 400 egg cells mature and leave the ovaries. The probabilities, then, that any given sperm or any given egg will grow into a reasoning adult human being are extraordinarily low even if pregnancy occurred with each ejaculation. And happily that does not happen!

Once a zygote is formed, however, the probability is relatively high that it will grow into an adult human being. How high that probability is depends on the rate of spontaneous abortion. The scientific community disagrees about just how high that rate is; some estimate as low as 15 percent, others as high as 50 percent.[9] Even if the higher estimate is correct, however, the probability that any given zygote will become an adult human being is very high when compared with the probability that any given sperm or egg will become part of such a being. And, the argument goes, a difference in probabilities makes a moral difference. If a person were to shoot into a bush and the chances were 200 million to one that in doing so another person would be killed, it is not very likely that the shooter would be held blameworthy for such an act. But if the chances were one in two that so shooting would kill a person, the shooter would be subject to moral censure. Differences in probabilities, then, make a moral difference, and so the conservative believes that this objection can be answered. Moreover, the conservative points out, the zygote has a complete human genetic code, whereas neither the sperm nor the egg does. Some have questioned, however, whether mere difference in genetic code is morally relevant.

Let us conclude this survey of the conservative position by noting some difficulties. The first problem to be discussed is unique to this particular instantiation of conservatism; the others are difficulties that all conservatives must address.

First, as already indicated, the eliminative strategy involves an inherent weakness. It is not possible to know whether all of the alternative views have been considered. Since the possibilities seem nearly endless, one can be reasonably sure that all possibilities have not been considered. In any case, a *positive* argument should be given for the thesis that the fetus is a person and so possesses moral rights from the moment of conception. Few positive arguments have been advanced in support of this thesis, however. Sometimes conservatives claim that mere membership in the species *Homo sapiens* is sufficient to the moral task. But something must be added to support such a view. Some will appeal to religion, claiming God has endowed all human beings with the right to life. Here we shall not consider such religious views, however, because there is hardly a consensus about what constitutes religious truths. Moreover, we are looking for philosophical grounds in support of the various positions.

Second, consider the case in which a woman becomes pregnant as a result of being raped. Many are inclined to approve of abortion under such circumstances. Yet it seems that the conservative cannot consistently allow for this. Recall that the essence of the conservative position is that fetuses possess the right to life, the same right to life as adult human beings. When rape takes place, obviously a serious wrong has occurred. But the wrongdoing has been perpetrated by the fetus's father, not by the fetus. When a person does something wrong, he sometimes forfeits certain rights. The fetus, however, cannot be said to have forfeited some of its rights because of the immoral actions of its father. The moral turpitude of the father cannot affect the fetus's right to life!

Conservatives, then, seemingly will be hard-pressed to permit abortion even when pregnancy is due to rape. Conservatives must bite the bullet, it seems, and argue that a woman must make a sacrifice for the sake of the fetus. Of course, in political contexts some conservatives *say* that they allow an exception in the case of pregnancy due to rape. But the issue is whether such an exception is *consistent* with their underlying assumption. It seems not.

Third, it is not even clear that conservatives can allow for abortion when the woman's life is at stake. Again, some conservatives *say* that they can consistently allow for abortion in this extreme and rare case. But can they? What we have in such a situation is a conflict of rights. The right to life of the woman conflicts with the right to life of the fetus. Some conservatives have suggested that in these extreme circumstances the woman's right to life may prevail because she has the right to defend herself. This is controversial, however. The being that poses a threat to the woman is innocent, and, as we shall discuss later, some doubt that killing innocent threats constitutes genuine self-defense. In any case, considerations of fairness may compel conservatives to prefer the fetus to the woman in situations of extreme conflict. After all, according to conservatives, each is innocent and each has the right to life. If one must be sacrificed and one saved, would it not be fairer to prefer the fetus because it has had no chance to experience life while the woman has had a number of years? Perhaps conservatives can avoid this consequence. But when the foundation of their view is that the fetus has an *equal* right to life, they must provide an argument to show how this result can be avoided.

A fourth difficulty is that conservatives must condemn as killing certain forms of birth control. In particular, any form of birth control that allows conception to take place but prevents implantation—such as an IUD (intrauterine device)—must be considered wrong because it destroys a being with the right to life. The same is true of RU 486. Is using an IUD or RU 486 really a form of impermissible killing? Perhaps they are, but certainly additional argument is needed to show this.

Fifth, conservatives must oppose all abortions chosen for eugenic reasons. In some cases, perhaps conservatives can convince us that they are protecting a class of individuals from acts of discrimination—for example, when a fetus is aborted because of the presence of Down's syndrome. But to hold this position in all cases seems implausible. Is it really wrong to abort an anencephalic fetus?

Finally, if abortion is the murder of an innocent person, one would expect conservatives to recommend penalties commensurate with such a wrong. But they are often silent on this topic. Some politicians are simply disingenuous, claiming that women who choose abortions are themselves victims and that doctors who perform the act should be punished. It is hard to see how a woman who understands her options and chooses to have an abortion is a victim. And it is hard to understand why conservatives are reticent to recommend commensurate punishment for her, other than the obvious fact that such a measure is unpopular.

The Liberal Position

Liberals on the abortion issue want to show that abortion is virtually always permissible if that is what the pregnant woman wants, but infanticide is wrong. Part of their task is the "line drawing problem": they must show that fetuses do not have the right to life. The other part of their task is to show why infanticide is wrong. Here we shall describe one of the better-known lines of argument for the liberal position, sketched by Mary Anne Warren.[10]

As Warren sees it, the crucial issue in abortion is defining the *moral community*—that is, the set of beings with full and equal moral rights. Conservatives hold that all human beings are members of the moral community. This position enables them to make a simple argument against abortion, which Warren sets out as follows:

1. **It is wrong to kill innocent human beings.**
2. **Fetuses are innocent human beings.**
3. **Therefore, it is wrong to kill fetuses.**

The trouble with this argument is that the term *human* can be used in two senses. *Human* in the moral sense means a full-fledged member of the moral community. *Human* in the genetic sense designates a member of the species *Homo sapiens*. In the conservatives' argument, premise 1 is defensible and avoids begging any questions about abortion only if *human* is used in the moral sense. Premise 2 is obviously true and avoids begging any questions about abortion only if *human* is used in the genetic sense. But the conclusion, line 3, follows from lines 1 and 2 only if *human* is used in the same sense. When an argument appears to be valid only because the same term is used to mean two different things, the argument is said to commit the *fallacy of equivocation*. So unless an argument can show that whatever is genetically human is also morally human, the original argument is flawed: either one of its premises begs the question on the issue of abortion or it commits the fallacy of equivocation.

Warren uses the term *person* (and *people*) to designate members of the moral community. Her task is to determine what characteristics a being must possess to be a person. She suggests that in formulating these characteristics, we engage in a thought experiment: ask ourselves how we would decide whether a totally alien being was a person. Warren suggests that the following traits are central to the concept of personhood: (1) consciousness, particularly the capacity to feel pain; (2) the developed capacity to reason; (3) self-motivated activity, relatively independent of genetic or external control; (4) the capacity to communicate complex messages; and (5) self-awareness and the presence of self-concepts.

Warren does not explain how she arrived at this list of traits, though one suspects that she has abstracted from the paradigm of an adult human being. She admits that she cannot formulate precise definitions of these criteria, and she says that we need not suppose that an entity must possess all of these attributes to be considered a person. Some combination of several of these traits may be sufficient for personhood. And perhaps no one of these traits is by itself necessary for personhood. However, these difficulties need not infect the discussion of abortion, because, according to Warren, human fetuses possess *none* of traits 1 through 5 and therefore certainly are not persons.

If traits 1 through 5 are the primary criteria of personhood, then clearly *genetic* humanity is neither necessary nor sufficient for establishing that an entity is a person with full moral rights. It is not sufficient because some genetic humans are not persons. Warren thinks that human fetuses are not persons, and presumably individuals in a persistent vegetative state and anencephalic infants are not either. Genetic humanity is not necessary, or at least not known to be necessary, because perhaps members of other species have all of the traits or the proper combination of them. Perhaps dolphins or chimpanzees qualify as persons; we cannot rule this out without investigation.

What is crucial to Warren's argument is her claim that human fetuses lack traits 1 through 5. On the basis of that, she asserts that no legal restrictions on the stage of pregnancy in which an abortion may be performed can be justified on grounds that we should protect the rights of fetuses. So unless there are other grounds for prohibiting the procedure, *no legal restrictions* should be placed on abortion.

This argument creates an obvious problem for Warren, however. Newborn infants are not significantly more personlike than late-stage fetuses. So Warren's argument appears to justify too much: not only will it permit abortion at any stage of fetal development, but it will permit infanticide too. Warren wants to avoid this consequence.[11] She admits that in her view infanticide does not constitute killing a person, but she claims that nevertheless it is more difficult to justify than abortion. The principal reason that infanticide is usually wrong in our society is that if a newborn's parents do not want it or cannot afford it, often other people are eager to adopt it and give it care. It would be wrong to deprive these others of a source of great happiness. So we have a utilitarian argument against infanticide. Even if an infant is virtually unadoptable—say, because of severe disabilities—Warren says that it would usually be wrong to kill it because most people would rather support public institutions that care for people with disabilities than allow them to be killed.

But if a utilitarian argument can be used to prohibit infanticide, it seems able also to be employed against late-stage abortions. After all, many are desperate to adopt a child and would gladly pay for the medical expenses of the pregnant woman. One can argue, as before, that it is wrong to deprive these people of such a great source of happiness.

Warren is aware of this potential problem and has a response. She claims that the utilitarian argument cannot be used to prohibit late-stage abortions because "a pregnant woman's right to protect her own life and health clearly outweighs other people's desire that the fetus be preserved."[12] But Warren's response here is not adequate. She contends that abortion at any stage of fetal development and for any reason should be permitted. To block the argument that appeals to the happiness of others and that she endorses against infanticide, Warren invokes a woman's right to protect her life and health. But what if neither of these factors is present? What if we have a late-stage pregnancy that is no threat to the woman's life or health? Then the utilitarian argument can be invoked to prohibit such abortions. So Warren's reply does not protect all cases of abortion from the utilitarian argument.

We conclude by noting several problems with Warren's position. First, she does not defend the set of criteria she lists for membership in the moral community. She seems to think that they are rather obvious and will be accepted by opponents of abortion too.[13] This is surely misplaced optimism, however. Perhaps these criteria can be defended. But in the absence of such a defense, one is left wondering whether they should be accepted.

Second, Warren says that it is clear that human fetuses possess none of traits 1 through 5. It is far from obvious, however, that late-stage fetuses do not possess consciousness, which Warren explains as "the capacity to feel pain." Surely third-trimester fetuses, at least, have the biological equipment needed to experience pain. Perhaps Warren means something different by "consciousness." If so, she needs to explain it; if not, she appears mistaken.

Third, Warren seems to make what might be called "the all-or-nothing assumption." She assumes that either human fetuses are beings with the full complement of moral rights, including the right to life, or they have no rights at all. But such an assumption seems dubious. Most people do not regard nonhuman animals as beings with the full complement of moral rights. Yet they do not think that people may do anything they wish to animals; torturing animals is wrong. And this is not merely an abstract point; it may well have application to abortions, especially ones performed late in pregnancy. For if at some point during pregnancy fetuses can experience pain, this condition would suggest that from that point on any form of abortion that inflicted pain on the fetus is prima facie wrong. And this rationale need not assume that the fetus has the right to life. Indeed, inflicting pain on a sentient being may be wrong even if that being has no rights at all.

Finally, as noted earlier, it is difficult to show that while abortion should always be permitted, infanticide may be prohibited. Warren's utilitarian argument against infanticide appears to apply equally well against at least some late-stage abortions.

Interlude: The Potentiality Principle

Our discussion of the conservative and liberal views omits one serious point of dispute between them. This concerns the moral relevance of potential. We can put this in the form of a question: What is the moral significance of the fact that human fetuses have the potential to become persons?

A *potential person* is a being that will become an actual person (that is, a being who will acquire all of the characteristics needed for personhood) in the normal course of its development. Those who believe that potentiality is morally important endorse the *potentiality principle:* any organism that will in the normal course of its development acquire the characteristics that endow a being with the right to life has a serious right to life now in virtue of that potentiality. This principle enables conservatives to defend their position. For human zygotes are potential persons; they will in the normal course of their development acquire the characteristics that adult human beings have. Because we believe that adult human beings have the right to life, the potentiality principle instructs us to assign the same right to life to fetuses.

Apart from the fact that it supports their position, conservatives have other reasons for endorsing the potentiality principle. First, this principle enables conservatives to defend their position without specifying what properties endow beings with the right to life. The idea is this. Virtually everyone agrees that adult human beings have the right to life. Whatever the properties are that endow them with this right, human fetuses possess those properties potentially; they will come to have them in the normal course of their development. This is an important advantage because given the widely divergent accounts provided by conservatives and liberals, you might reasonably doubt that this dispute will ever be resolved. Yet conservatives and liberals alike agree that adult human beings have the right to life. So, if they also accept the potentiality principle, the debate about abortion can apparently be resolved without addressing the seemingly intractable issue of what properties endow a being with the right to life.

A second reason for endorsing the potentiality principle is that it provides conservatives with a secular basis for their position. This is not meant to be an antireligious statement. Rather, in the United States, public policy is not supposed to be made on the basis of religious principles. Too often, however, conservatives have defended their position by appealing to the tenets of particular religions. The potentiality principle is not linked to any particular religion and, if plausible, can be accepted by all.

Third, neither conservatives nor liberals object to "tampering" with fetuses of other species. For example, pig fetuses are often used for instructional purposes in introductory biology classes. Yet we might ask what the moral difference is between a pig fetus in its early stage of development and a human fetus in its early stage of development. The difference, surely, is not in what they are *now* but rather in what they can become. And that consideration suggests that potentiality is morally relevant.

Finally, if we value and promote, say, rationality as it is exhibited by adult human beings, then it may seem odd not to value beings that are potentially rational as well. So, conservatives have good reasons to accept the potentiality principle (though whether the ascription of rights follows from the fact that we value something is doubtful). Indeed, some think that this is the best basis for defending the conservative view.

Liberals and moderates alike have been critical of the potentiality principle. Here we shall sketch only a few representative criticisms of it.

First, let us consider a criticism of the potentiality principle advanced by Warren.[14] She is willing to grant that potentiality is important and that there may be a strong prima facie reason for not destroying potential persons. But, she contends, even if a potential person has a prima facie right to life, "such a right could not possibly outweigh the right of a woman to obtain an abortion, because the rights of any actual person invariably outweigh those of any potential person."

Realizing that this claim is not obvious, Warren provides a defense. She asks us to imagine that a space explorer falls into the hands of an alien culture. Scientists in this culture have perfected the technique of cloning, and they decide to create a few hundred thousand humans by breaking up the explorer's body and using the component cells to generate fully developed human beings. Warren says that in this case the explorer has every right to escape and thereby deprive all of these potential people of their potential lives because the explorer's right to life outweighs all of theirs together. Warren adds that the explorer would have the right to escape even if it were not his life that the alien scientists planned to take, but only nine months of his freedom, or even one day. Warren even thinks that the explorer would have a right to escape if he had been caught as a result of his own carelessness, or even if he got caught deliberately. Warren apparently thinks that these examples are uncontroversial. If she is correct, then she has shown that the rights of actual persons always outweigh the rights of potential persons. And if this is correct, then the rights of a pregnant woman will always outweigh the rights of the fetus. This argument will so weaken the potentiality principle as to make it useless in the defense of conservativism.

A second criticism of the potentiality principle is advanced by Michael Tooley.[15] The moral symmetry principle is an assumption on which this criticism is based. According to the *moral symmetry principle*, if the motivation is the same, then there is no moral difference between intentionally refraining from bringing about state of affairs S and actively preventing state of affairs S from occurring. Similarly, the moral symmetry principle tells us that, if the motivation is the same, then there is no moral difference in the action of a person who brings about state of affairs S and one who refrains from preventing S from occurring.

Defenders of this principle usually try to render it plausible by giving examples. Consider the following two cases. First, suppose that Gomez sees that Kowalski will be killed by a bomb unless he warns her. But because Gomez wants Kowalski dead, he does nothing and allows her to be killed by the bomb. Now suppose that Gomez wants Kowalski dead and so shoots her. Do we think that Gomez's behavior is less reprehensible in the first case than the second? Defenders of the moral symmetry principle think that we do not, and a plausible explanation of why we do not is that we accept the moral symmetry principle.

Given this, Tooley now asks us to consider the following situation. Suppose that we have discovered a special chemical with very unusual properties. When injected into the brain of a kitten, this chemical will cause the kitten to develop into a cat that possesses the same sort of brain that human beings possess. Cats that have been injected can think, use language, express their desires, indicate their worries about the future, and the like. How should such cats be treated? Concerning this hypothetical case, Tooley makes four important points:

1. If the right to life is ascribed to adult members of the species *Homo sapiens*, then consistency requires that the right to life be ascribed to cats that have undergone the process of development resulting from the injection with the special chemical. There are no morally relevant differences between adult human beings and these extraordinary cats. Differences in physical appearance are obvious, but these are morally insignificant.

2. It would not be wrong to refrain from injecting a kitten with this special chemical and to kill it instead. (This assumes that kittens do not have the right to life. You can select some other nonhuman animal if you disagree about the status of kittens. What is important is that a being can be transformed into one with the right to life.) The mere fact that it is within our power to transform a kitten into a being that possesses the right to life does not imply that we have an obligation to do so. If a normal kitten does not possess the right to life, we have no duty to change it into a being that does have this right. If there were such an obligation, all forms of birth control would be wrong, and reproduction may be obligatory.

3. The moral symmetry principle tells us that if it is not wrong to refrain from initiating a given causal process, then it is not wrong to interfere with such a process before the end has been brought about. Thus, if it is not wrong to refrain from injecting a kitten with the special chemical and to kill it instead, then it is not wrong to inject the kitten with the special chemical but kill it before it develops the properties that endow a being with the right to life. In the former case, a person is refraining from initiating a certain process; in the latter case, that person is preventing the process from reaching its completion. This result follows from the moral symmetry principle and the conclusion reached in point 2.

4. If it is not wrong to kill an injected kitten before it develops the properties that endow a being with the right to life, then neither is it wrong to kill a member of the species *Homo sapiens* that does not now possess those properties but will acquire them if allowed to develop. An injected kitten and a human fetus have the same moral status: neither presently has the properties necessary to endow a being with the right to life, but each will come to possess them if allowed to develop. If potentiality endows a being with the right to life, then both the injected kitten and human fetuses possess the right to life, and it would be wrong to kill either. But, as was argued, it is not wrong to kill an injected kitten. Therefore, it is not wrong to kill a member of the species *Homo sapiens* before it develops the properties that give a being the right to life.

Thus, Tooley claims to have refuted the potentiality principle. And if conservatives must adopt this principle, then their position too has been refuted. No attempt to evaluate this argument will be made here. The reader should be aware, however, that this criticism presupposes the correctness of the moral symmetry principle, and many have doubted its plausibility. To mention just one criticism, some wonder whether agents' motivations are ever relevant to determining the rightness or wrongness of their ensuing actions. Defenders of moral symmetry seem to assume that motivations do affect the moral status of actions, which is not obviously correct.

Both Warren and Tooley try to refute the potentiality principle by constructing counterexamples. In both cases, the counterexamples depend on hypothetical cases that you might say have been imported from science fiction. If you are like many people, you have little patience with this approach and wonder why realistic examples are not used. But there is a reason for this. The only obvious examples of potential persons that we have are human fetuses, and they cannot be used to assess the potentiality principle because the debate about abortion concerns their moral status. Thus, different examples are needed. Because they are not readily available in the real world, hypothetical cases must be constructed.

These first two criticisms of the potentiality principle try to show that it is false. A third set of criticisms has a more modest aim, namely, to show that this principle does not fit completely well with the overall conservative position.[16] Two points in particular lead one to wonder whether conservatives can, after all, endorse the potentiality principle. First, not all human fetuses have the potential to develop all of the morally significant properties possessed by adult human beings. Severely defective fetuses lack this potential and so will not be accorded the right to life in virtue of potential. One suspects that this will not sit well with conservatives. Second, the principle may prove more than the conservative wants; for it appears that human sex cells, gametes, also have potential. And if they do, conservatives must also favor the prohibition of birth control. Whether the sperm and egg have this potential depends in part on how we are to understand the normal course of development. If it is merely a statistical notion, then individual sperm and individual eggs do not have potential in this sense. But conservatives usually insist that the notion is not statistical,[17] and for good reason; if it were a statistical notion and if the rate of spontaneous abortion is higher than previously supposed, human fetuses too will lack potential in this sense. Conservatives must avoid this last consequence; but if they can do so only by ascribing the same potential, and therefore the same moral status, to gametes as to fetuses, perhaps they should just abandon the potentiality principle.

Full evaluation of the potentiality principle will not be undertaken here. It is important, however, especially because it promises to provide conservatives with a secular basis for their position.

Moderates

Moderates on the abortion issue encompass a wide range of positions. They may vary in both the reasons allowed to justify abortion and the stage of fetal development beyond which abortion may not occur. Several versions of the moderate view will be examined.

Surveying the literature on abortion, one cannot help but be pessimistic that any consensus will emerge about what properties endow a being with the right to life. The disagreements on this issue appear to be fundamental. Exactly why this is so is not clear; perhaps the argument proceeds too quickly without an appropriate analysis of rights. In any case, if this issue cannot be resolved, no progress can be made. But perhaps this pessimism is not warranted. One version of the moderate position does not try to determine what properties are necessary for possessing the right to life or when fetuses acquire such a right. Instead, a different tact is taken.[18] This version attempts to establish two claims: (1) even if the fetus is a person with the right to life, it does not follow that abortion is always wrong; and (2) even if the fetus is not a person and does not have the right to life, it does not follow that abortion is always permissible. We shall examine how each of these claims might be established and what the resulting policy on abortion will be. Our discussion of claim 1 will be quite extensive.

If claim 1 can be established, that achievement will be quite significant. Conservatives and liberals alike have assumed that if it is shown that the fetus has the right to life, then it will follow that abortion is wrong. What defenders of claim 1 hope to show is that such an inference is unwarranted. If claim 1 can be defended, this will damage the conservative position; for the conservative's most cherished premise will have been granted, yet it will have been shown that abortion is not always wrong. (As we shall see, establishing claim 2 will damage the liberal position.)

In defending claim 1, we will consider three different approaches.

The first approach appeals to the notion of self-defense. Suppose that carrying the fetus to term will endanger the life of the woman. The woman is a person with the right to life, and she has a right to defend herself when her life is endangered. So, even if the fetus does have the right to life, the woman is permitted to abort it if doing so is necessary to save her own life. This argument, if successful, only shows that abortion is permissible in a relatively rare type of case. But its purpose is modest: to show that the assumption that it is always wrong to kill a being with the right to life is false.

Some wonder whether this first approach even accomplishes its modest aim. The problem lies in unraveling the concept of self-defense. In a paradigmatic case of self-defense, you kill X because X is trying to kill you, and killing X is the only way to prevent X from killing you. In such a case, X is a threat to you and X is culpable. But sometimes a person who is a threat to your life may be innocent. Consider this example. Someone has rigged the light switch so that when it is moved it will set off a bomb in the room you now occupy. Y, an innocent person, is about to move the switch and thus detonate the bomb unwittingly. You can prevent Y from detonating the bomb only if you shoot Y. Y is an innocent threat to you. Does self-defense justify killing an innocent threat? The relevance to the debate about abortion, of course, is that when the fetus is a threat to the life of the woman, it is an innocent threat.

Some think that if a crazed child or a hypnotized person were attacking you and you could save your life only by killing your attacker, then this is a legitimate case of self-defense. Nothing in the notion of self-defense implies that the threat must be culpable. Matters are complicated even further because women do not typically perform abortions on themselves; third parties are involved. We cannot hope to resolve the debate about the concept of self-defense here. Suffice it to say that *if* killing an innocent threat constitutes a legitimate case of self-defense, and *if* third parties may provide assistance in these cases, then this first approach establishes claim 1 for a very limited number of cases.

A second approach for establishing claim 1 appeals to the notion of a supererogatory act. A supererogatory act is morally desirable but not required; it is above and beyond the call of duty. Actions that involve great sacrifice on the part of their agents are typically, though not always, thought to be supererogatory. If one person saved the life of another at the expense of her own life, we would say in most circumstances that she had performed a supererogatory act. Because supererogatory acts are not required, one is permitted to refrain from performing such acts. A person who refuses to perform a supererogatory act cannot be accused of wrong-doing because of that refusal.

Now consider the situation in which carrying the fetus to term will endanger the woman's life. Even if the fetus possesses the right to life, a woman is not required to sacrifice her own life to save another; if she were to do so, the act would be supererogatory. So, in such cases, a woman is permitted not to carry the fetus to term. And this second approach may not be limited merely to cases where the woman's life is threatened by continuing the pregnancy. For it may well be the case that other sorts of sacrifices involved in carrying the fetus to term will render such an act supererogatory. Examples might include when carrying the fetus to term will produce great emotional trauma (as when pregnancy was due to rape), when having a child would be a great financial burden, and the like.

The point of this second approach is this: even if the fetus has the right to life, aborting it is not wrong in those cases where completing the pregnancy would be a supererogatory act. Of course, disagreement is apt to arise about which of those cases are properly regarded as supererogatory.

A third approach for establishing claim 1 says that we must examine more carefully just what is involved with the right to life. To put it another way, this approach asks what it is that the right to life gives one a right to. To understand this approach, we need to reiterate some of the earlier remarks about rights. Rights have associated with them correlative duties. If you have a right, someone else has a duty regarding you. For example, if you have a right to this book because you purchased it, everyone else has a duty not to steal it, not to write in it without your permission, and so forth. These duties on others are correlative with your property right.

Rights can be either positive or negative. A *positive right* has associated with it positive duties, that is, duties to provide the right holder with goods, services, and the like. If children have a right to be educated, this puts duties on some others to provide them with various services. A *negative right* has associated with it negative duties, that is, duties that others have to refrain from doing certain things to the right holder. Property rights are usually understood as negative. Your property rights put duties on others not to do certain things, at least not without your permission.

The right to life might be understood as either a positive right or a negative right. We must explain these two interpretations and then ask which is more plausible. If the right to life is positive, then it gives the possessor of that right a claim against others that they provide her whatever is necessary to maintain life, short of seriously risking their own lives. By contrast, if the right to life is negative, this gives its possessor a claim against others that they not kill her unjustly.[19] According to the negative interpretation, others properly respect a person's right to life if they refrain from doing certain things; they have no positive duties because of another's right to life.

How should the right to life be construed? Is it better understood as a positive right or a negative right? This third approach to establishing claim 1 says that the negative construal of the right to life is more plausible. Why? If the right to life is understood as a positive right, unacceptable consequences follow. Consider this case. Suppose that Furillo has a fatal form of leukemia, and only a bone marrow transplant will save his life. Furillo is difficult to match, and as it turns out you are the only suitable donor. You are not related to Furillo and do not know him. If the right to life requires others to do whatever is necessary to maintain another's life, then you are required to donate bone marrow to Furillo; if you fail to do so, you violate his right to life. But this result seems absurd. Certainly it would be very nice of you to donate bone marrow to Furillo. But to say that you are required to do so seems doubtful; to say that you violate Furillo's right to life by failing to do so seems ludicrous. Indeed, if you were to donate bone marrow to Furillo, this would be an act of Good Samaritanism, and in the United States Good Samaritanism is normally not legally required.

This point about American law is illustrated in a case involving cousins, Robert McFall and David Shimp.[20] In June 1978, McFall was diagnosed as having aplastic anemia, a usually fatal disease in which the patient's bone marrow fails to produce enough red and white blood cells and platelets. McFall's only hope of survival was to receive a bone marrow transplant. His six siblings were examined, but none was compatible to serve as a donor. Then McFall's first cousin, David Shimp, underwent preliminary tests, and he was determined to be a perfect match for tissue compatibility. At that point, however, Shimp refused to undergo further tests and withdrew as a potential donor. Reasons for his refusal were not entirely clear, though apparently the requests of his wife and mother and a longtime family feud were factors in the decision. Many people tried to persuade Shimp to change his mind, but he would not. McFall then filed suit to compel Shimp to undergo a bone marrow transplant. Pennsylvania (Allegheny County) Judge John Flaherty ruled against McFall. Judge

Flaherty said that although Shimp's refusal to donate was morally indefensible, nevertheless there is no legal duty to take action to save
another's life and certainly no duty to undergo a transplant for the sake
of another. Robert McFall died on August 10, 1978.[21]

Compelling a woman to continue pregnancy, then, would be a rare
case of compulsory Good Samaritanism and unfair. The only other such
cases in the United States are ones that involve persons with special skills,
such as health care practitioners, who may be required to render medical
assistance at the scene of an accident.

The right to life, then, is commonly understood as negative. But what
are the consequences of this observation for abortion? The right to life
gives one a right not to be killed unjustly. As the case of McFall and
Shimp shows, the right to life does not give one a right to use the body of
another person. One has the right to use another person's body only
when that other person has *given* one such a right. So even if the fetus has
the right to life, it does not have the right to the continued use of the
woman's body unless the woman has given it such a right. If the woman
has not given the fetus the right to use her body, she may abort it if she
wishes. (Notice, however, that having the right to abort the fetus is not
the same as having the right to kill it. Should an aborted fetus be alive, the
woman will have no right to kill it.)

Cases where it is plausible to say that a woman has *not* given the fetus
the right to use her body include when pregnancy is due to rape and
when the woman took reasonable precautions to avoid pregnancy by using a reliable method of birth control. On the other hand, if the woman
engages in sexual intercourse voluntarily, uses no method of birth control, and wants to become pregnant, then arguably she *has* given the fetus
the right to use her body. Even if these are clear cases, undoubtedly many
borderline situations are possible where it is not clear whether the
woman has given the fetus the right to use her body. But borderline cases
aside, this third approach, if successful, provides a defense of claim 1 that
covers far more situations than the first two approaches.

This third approach forces us to confront the issue of how properly to
understand the right to life. The example of the bone marrow donor certainly suggests that the positive interpretation of the right to life is too
strong. And if that case does not convince you, suppose that one person
needed one of another person's kidneys to live; surely in this case failure
to give does not violate the would-be recipient's right to life, even though
one can donate without serious risk to one's own life. On the other hand,
the negative interpretation of the right to life seems too weak in certain
cases. Suppose that you encounter an abandoned infant in the woods on
a cold night. This infant has the right to life. But if that is merely a right

not to be killed unjustly, then you cannot be said to have wronged the infant if you refuse to bring it to safety. This seems wrong; it seems to make the right to life virtually useless.

At least two different responses might be made here that would allow us to retain the negative interpretation of the right to life. First, one might say that refusing to help the infant is just a way of killing it. The problem here is that this could be extended to many cases involving adults too, and thus the differences between the positive and negative construals of the right to life would vanish. Second, and more plausibly, one might argue that if you refused to help the abandoned infant, you would be guilty of wrongdoing, though not guilty of violating its right to life; not all wrongdoing must violate rights.

At the very least, this third approach challenges us to make clearer exactly what the right to life is and what it guarantees its possessors.

This defense of claim 1 pulls us away from the conservative view. If successful, it shows that the fetus's possession of the right to life does not always preclude abortion. Claim 2, if established, will pull us away from the liberal position by showing that abortion is not always permissible even if the fetus lacks the right to life. Our examination of claim 2 will be rather brief.

Beings with the right to life get full moral consideration; they are persons with a rich complement of moral rights. But it does not follow from the fact that a being is not a person, that we may do anything we wish to that being. To assume this would be to commit oneself to what was earlier called the all-or-nothing assumption, which is surely false. Within our own legal system, nonhuman animals seem to have some but not full moral status. Torturing animals is wrong, and not just because it might offend other people; it is wrong because of its effects on the animals. Killing animals merely for the fun of it may be wrong too. On the other hand, most people eat meat and so apparently approve of killing animals for food. This position suggests that animals deserve some but not full moral consideration. Obviously the moral status of animals is a hotly debated topic, one we certainly cannot resolve here. But if we take this position as representing a serious possibility, it has ramifications for claim 2.

Even if the human fetus is not a person with the full complement of rights, it need not follow that it has no rights at all. Like animals, the fetus may have some moral status. If, for example, at some point in its development the fetus is capable of experiencing pain, then it may at least have a right not to have pain inflicted on it gratuitously. We shall discuss this point later, but for now we can see that abortion might be wrong even if the fetus lacks the right to life. For some forms of abortion at certain points of fetal development may inflict pain on the fetus, which at least provides a moral reason against the procedure. The more abstract point is simply this: merely establishing that the fetus lacks the right to life does not automatically resolve the debate about abortion. One would also have to establish that the fetus has *no* moral status, which is a much stronger and more difficult to defend claim.

To the extent that claims 1 and 2 are credible, we have good reason to be suspicious of the extreme views on the issue of abortion. Admittedly, however, merely establishing these two claims does not mark out a precise position. It leaves room for much argument about where to draw the moral lines.

Let us consider another version of the moderate position. This version attempts to incorporate two widely shared beliefs into a coherent position on abortion. (1) There is something about the fetus itself, and not merely the social consequences, that makes the practice of abortion morally problematic. (2) Late abortions are more difficult to justify from the moral point of view than early abortions. Many on whom the label "moderate" is properly placed will accept beliefs 1 and 2. But how might these two beliefs be justified?

Some moderates try to argue that the fetus becomes a person with the right to life some time after conception but before birth. Taking this approach requires one to specify the point at which fetuses obtain the right to life and to explain what traits generate such a right only then but not sooner. Because fetal development is continuous, it is difficult to see how there can be some magical point at which rights commence. Thus, this approach seems unpromising.

Recently, however, Edward Langerak has advanced a novel defense of the moderate position.[22] This argument combines two approaches more commonly associated with other positions. Langerak wants to account for beliefs 1 and 2 without stipulating at what point fetuses become persons with the right to life. To account for belief 1, Langerak appeals to a weakened version of the potentiality principle. To defend belief 2, he employs what has been called "the conferred claims approach." Let us examine this strategy briefly.

The weakened version of the potentiality principle may be stated as follows: If, in the normal course of its development, a being will come to have a person's claim to life, then by virtue of that fact the being has some claim to life. This principle attributes differential moral statuses to actual and potential persons. Actual persons have a full-fledged claim to life, as strong a claim as any beings have. Potential persons have some claim to life, but not as strong as actual persons. Normal human fetuses are potential persons, and so they have some claim to life. If a being has a claim to life, then killing it requires justification.

This version of the potentiality principle is weaker than the one discussed earlier. The stronger version of this principle gives potential persons the same moral status as actual persons. The weaker version gives potential persons some moral status, but not that equal to actual persons. Killing a potential person is not a morally neutral act; it requires justification. But it is easier to justify killing potential persons than actual persons. Exactly what sort of justification would permit killing a potential person but not an actual person is not always clear, however.

Why should the weaker version of the potentiality principle be accepted? Certainly it is more plausible than the stronger version. Potential persons do not seem to merit the same moral status as actual persons, though potentiality does seem to have some moral force. Humans are regarded as temporal beings, considering their pasts and probable futures nearly as much as the present. Notice that nearly as much respect is shown for presidents-elect and former presidents as is shown for the current president. And accepting the weakened version of the potentiality principle will explain why many have qualms about experiments performed on human fetuses but no similar reservations concerning experiments done on fetuses of other species. If the potentiality principle is plausible, then it provides support for belief 1. All abortions are, to some degree, morally problematic because they involve killing a potential person, and such beings have some claim to life. Something about the fetus itself—namely, its potential—makes abortion an act for which moral justification is required.

But the potentiality principle cannot account for belief 2, that late abortions are more problematic morally than early abortions. Whether a human fetus was just conceived or has been developing for eight months, it is still a potential person. A different approach is needed to establish the second belief. It should be pointed out, however, that the weaker potentiality principle is consistent with belief 2, though the stronger version is not. That is, it is compatible with the weaker version that the claims to life held by different potential people can vary in strength. Langerak employs the conferred claims approach to explain why the claim to life held by very young human fetuses is weaker than the claim to life of much more developed human fetuses. Langerak is even willing to admit that a neonate does not satisfy all of the necessary and sufficient conditions for being an actual person. But certainly society wants to assign to neonates a very strong claim to life, with good reasons for doing so. Support for conferring a much stronger claim to life to neonates and late-stage fetuses than to early-stage fetuses is based on an appeal to the consequences. Infants are so similar to young persons, according to this argument, that permitting infanticide would create a moral climate in which the legitimate claims of young persons would be endangered. By comparable reasoning, older fetuses are so similar to infants that allowing the former to be killed would endanger the lives of the latter. So, if society is to protect the lives of very young persons, it has good reasons for conferring on infants and older fetuses a very strong claim to life, a claim almost as strong as is possessed by actual persons.

To go to the other end of the spectrum, preventing the implantation of zygotes would surely have virtually no effect on how young persons, neonates, or older fetuses are treated. So the claim to life of the zygote before implantation is very weak. This approach allows moderates to agree with liberals that personhood is not achieved until after birth. Even so, appealing to the social consequences gives society good reason to allow the claim to life to vary in strength throughout development. It is weakest at conception and strongest at birth. And one might hold, as Langerak does, that its strength increases at certain natural points in pregnancy, such as implantation, quickening, and viability. As fetuses develop, they are becoming more like persons.

If this approach is accepted, then abortions during early stages of pregnancy will be permissible for almost any reason. Certainly the use of IUDs and RU 486 to prevent implantation will be permissible, even though each destroys a zygote. Or at least these will be uncontroversially permissible for a multitude of reasons, including if the pregnant woman is too young, if pregnancy is due to rape, and if having a child will be a physical or mental burden. At later stages, however, far fewer reasons will justify abortions. After viability, this approach will probably permit abortions only when the woman's life or physical health will be imperiled if pregnancy is continued, a rare situation. At this stage the fetus's claim to life is very strong, though not so strong as to require an actual person to put her own life at risk. Presumably no reason will justify infanticide, and infant euthanasia will be permissible only if adult euthanasia is too. The details of this approach must be worked out, but the idea is to present a graduated approach not predicated on the assumption that the fetus attains personhood.

A full evaluation of this position will focus on two points. First, the weakened version of the potentiality principle must be assessed. The idea behind it is to assign to fetuses some moral status without putting them on a par with normal adult human beings. Second, the empirical assertions employed in the application of the conferred claims approach must be examined. Is it really true, for example, that if the lives of older fetuses are taken at will, this practice will endanger the lives of neonates and young persons? True, it is difficult to determine when a neonate becomes a person, and so permitting the killing of neonates might well result in the killings of persons. But if, as is claimed, infants are not yet persons, then neither are older fetuses. It might then be recommended that we treat birth as a morally significant event. For we are sure that before birth we are not killing a person. In any case, a full evaluation will not be provided here.

One other version of the moderate position should be discussed very briefly. This approach, advanced by L. W. Sumner, courageously does try to draw the line.[23] This version of the moderate position is presented within the utilitarian framework. Utilitarianism, you will recall, is the theory that says that an agent ought to perform that action that produces consequences at least as good on balance for all affected parties as the consequences of any other act available to the agent. But to apply this theory to abortion (or any other issue), we must know who counts as affected parties. What does it take to have *moral standing?* Or, in language introduced earlier, what does it take to qualify to be a member of the moral community?

Although we cannot reconstruct Sumner's complete argument here, he defends sentience as the property that qualifies beings for moral standing. *Sentience* is the ability to experience sensations of pleasure and pain. Developed sentient beings have wants, aims, and desires, which can be either satisfied or frustrated. Because feelings are states of mind, sentient beings must be conscious. So far as we can determine, plant species and many animal species are not sentient. Sentience admits of degrees; some creatures are more sentient than others. Sumner argues that the transmission of pain requires mechanisms present only in beings with a central nervous system, and so the capacity for pleasure and pain is not possessed by invertebrate animals.

Because sentience is a matter of degree, it will lead to a graded moral standing; the greater a degree of sentience, the greater a being counts morally. But all sentient beings count for something. A criterion of sentience allows for the gradual emergence of moral standing. No moral issues arise directly in our interactions with inanimate objects. Because what is essential to moral standing is the capacity to suffer, moral standing can be lost (say, due to an irreversibly comatose state) or never gained at all (say, by an anencephalic infant).

If moral standing depends on sentience, then human fetuses gain moral standing when they acquire the capacity to experience pleasure and pain. When this occurs obviously depends on knowledge of the development of human fetuses, particularly the various parts of the brain. Sumner argues that the available evidence suggests that first-trimester fetuses are not yet sentient and that third-trimester fetuses are.[24] Sentience, he says, emerges some time during the second trimester, but exactly when is still not clear. This means that there will be indeterminate cases, but that possibility is not necessarily a weakness. A moral theory should not draw sharp lines where they do not exist or where human knowledge is too limited to know where they should be drawn.

Still, Sumner's position enables us to formulate an abortion policy based on principle. First-trimester fetuses have not yet attained moral standing, and so a decision about whether to terminate pregnancy at that stage is a private one to be made by the woman. Third-trimester fetuses have attained moral standing, and so abortions at this stage terminate the lives of beings with moral standing. This position does not mean that all such abortions should be prohibited, but it does mean that abortions should be permitted only when there are strong moral reasons for them. Sumner suggests that the only reasons that would justify late-term abortions are therapeutic (when the woman's well-being is in serious jeopardy) and eugenic (when the fetus will be severely deformed). Given the inevitable indeterminacy, where exactly to draw the line during the second trimester is not clear. Reasonable people can disagree here, and different societies can adopt different policies. But, according to Sumner's position, no society should proscribe first-trimester abortions, and no society should permit third-trimester abortions except for morally compelling reasons.

No attempt to evaluate Sumner's position will be made here. We should point out, however, that if one accepts the utilitarian framework, then a strong argument can be made that drawing the line at sentience is not arbitrary. For it is surely correct to say that beings that can suffer have a good of their own that can be promoted. And it is hard to see how the interests of any such being can be nonarbitrarily excluded from the utilitarian calculus. If this is correct, then at least some moderates have the conceptual resources to "draw the line" without being open to the charge of arbitrariness.

RECENT DEVELOPMENTS

Two recent works on abortion—by Peter Wenz and Ronald Dworkin—have defended a woman's right to choose abortion during the first two trimesters of pregnancy. But Wenz thinks that it is ill advised to rely on the right of privacy, and Dworkin says that it is a mistake to focus on whether the fetus is a person. Wenz argues for the right to choose by appealing to the right of religious freedom. Dworkin urges that we see the debate about abortion as spiritual and argues that the power of states to dictate how their citizens must respect the inherent value of life is limited.

These approaches place the debate about abortion in the realm of political philosophy and constitutional reasoning, and they are important. To pursue them here would take us somewhat far afield. But readers interested in these approaches will find these works stimulating.

SUMMARY

The abortion issue is unique because the extreme views—the conservative and liberal positions—often seem more plausible than their moderate competitors. The reason for this is that many reduce the debate about abortion to this choice: either fetuses possess the right to life from the moment of conception and therefore abortion is always wrong, or humans do not acquire the right to life until at least birth and therefore abortion is always permissible. Examining these two extreme views forces us to ask what properties endow beings with the right to life. Some who defend the conservative position believe that fetuses possess the right to life from the moment of conception because of genetic endowment. By contrast, liberals argue that properties such as the capacity for self-awareness and rationality are morally crucial and that human fetuses lack these. As we have seen, however, conservatives can grant these points if they can defend a strong version of the potentiality principle. Armed with such a principle, the conservative position can be defended without reverting to genetic endowment or divine conferral as the properties that give fetuses the right to life. Assessing this principle, therefore, is important in the debate about abortion.

The abortion issue entails more than this, however. As we saw in examining the moderate position, even if human fetuses have the right to life, it may not follow that abortion is always wrong. The assumption that this does follow is too simplistic, and the moderate forces us to think more clearly about how properly to understand the right to life. Moderates also challenge the assumption that if human fetuses do not have the right to life, then abortion is always permissible. Beings that do not have the full-fledged right to life can still have some moral status, and some human fetuses may fit this category. Other moderates invite us to consider the social consequences of allowing late-stage abortions, including the possibility that this will create a moral climate adverse to the rights of actual persons. Finally, some moderates argue that the criterion for moral standing is sentience and that human fetuses acquire this property some time during the second trimester of development. According to this view, early abortions are permissible, but late-stage abortions should be allowed only in extreme circumstances.

The principal questions concerning the abortion debate, then, are these: What properties are necessary for beings to possess the right to life? Do human fetuses, at any stage of their development, possess these properties? Does the fact that fetuses will come to possess these properties in the natural course of their development give them some moral status? And under what conditions is it permissible to kill a being that possesses the right to life?

Suggestions for Further Reading

Devine, Philip E. *The Ethics of Homicide* (Ithaca, NY: Cornell University Press, 1978).

Dworkin, Ronald. *Life's Dominion* (New York: Knopf, 1993).

English, Jane. "Abortion and the Concept of a Person." In Joel Feinberg, *The Problem of Abortion*, 2d ed. (Belmont, CA: Wadsworth, 1984), pp. 151–160.

Feinberg, Joel (ed.) *The Problem of Abortion*, 2d ed. (Belmont, CA: Wadsworth, 1984).

Langerak, Edward A. "Abortion: Listening to the Middle." In John Arras and Nancy Rhoden (eds.), *Ethical Issues in Modern Medicine*, 3d ed. (Mountain View, CA: Mayfield, 1989), pp. 286–292.

Marquis, Don. "Why Abortion Is Immoral." *Journal of Philosophy*, Vol. 86 (1989), pp. 183–202.

Munson, Ronald (ed.). *Intervention and Reflection: Basic Issues in Medical Ethics*, 4th ed. (Belmont, CA: Wadsworth, 1992), Chapter 1.

Noonan, John T., Jr. "An Almost Absolute Value in History." In Ronald Munson (ed.), *Intervention and Reflection: Basic Issues in Medical Ethics*, 4th ed. (Belmont, CA: Wadsworth, 1992), pp. 67–72.

Sumner, L. W. "Abortion." In Donald VanDeVeer and Tom Regan (eds.), *Health Care Ethics* (Philadelphia: Temple University Press, 1987), pp. 162–183.

Sumner, L. W. *Abortion and Moral Theory* (Princeton, NJ: Princeton University Press, 1981).

Thomson, Judith Jarvis. "A Defense of Abortion." In Joel Feinberg (ed.), *The Problem of Abortion*, 2d ed. (Belmont, CA: Wadsworth, 1984), pp. 173–187.

Warren, Mary Anne. "On the Moral and Legal Status of Abortion." In Joel Feinberg (ed.), *The Problem of Abortion*, 2d ed. (Belmont, CA: Wadsworth, 1984), pp. 102–119.

Wenz, Peter. *Abortion Rights as Religious Freedom* (Philadelphia: Temple University Press, 1992).

Notes

1. This way of putting the question is suggested by Roger Wertheimer in "Understanding the Abortion Argument," in Joel Feinberg (ed.), *The Problem of Abortion*, 2d ed. (Belmont, CA: Wadsworth, 1984), p. 43.

2. The labels for the first four sets of reasons discussed here are suggested in L. W. Sumner, "Abortion," in Donald VanDeVeer and Tom Regan (eds.), *Health Care Ethics* (Philadelphia: Temple University Press, 1987), p. 167.

3. For a discussion of the topic of abortion for the purposes of gender selection, see "Prenatal Diagnosis for Sex Choice," *Hastings Center Report*, Vol. 10 1980), pp. 15–20, and Holly Smith Goldman, "Amniocentesis for Sex Selection," in Marc D. Basson (ed.), *Ethics, Humanism, and Medicine* (New York: Liss, 1980), pp. 81–93.

4. Justice Harry Blackmun is the author of the majority opinion in *Roe v. Wade*, reprinted in Ronald Munson (ed.), *Intervention and Reflection: Basic Issues in Medical Ethics*, 4th ed. (Belmont, CA: Wadsworth, 1992), pp. 61–67.

5. The version of the conservative position presented here (including most of the criticisms of the other positions) is defended by John T. Noonan, Jr., "An Almost Absolute Value in History," in Ronald Munson (ed.), *Intervention and Reflection: Basic Issues in Medical Ethics*, 4th ed. (Belmont, CA: Wadsworth, 1992), pp. 67–72. In a few cases, changes in the argument have been made.

6. Noonan, "An Almost Absolute Value in History," p. 68.

7. Those who adhere strictly to Catholic theology hold that it is wrong to practice birth control. They do *not* base their position, however, on the belief that the sperm and egg have the right to life.

8. See especially Noonan, "An Almost Absolute Value in History," p. 70.

9. See Edward A. Langerak, "Abortion: Listening to the Middle," *Hastings Center Report*, Vol. 9 (1979), p. 26.

10. Mary Anne Warren, "On the Moral and Legal Status of Abortion," in Feinberg, *The Problem of Abortion*, pp. 102–119.

11. Some who argue for a more radical position believe that infanticide, too, should be permitted. See Michael Tooley, "A Defense of Abortion and Infanticide," in Joel Feinberg (ed.), *The Problem of Abortion* (Belmont, CA: Wadsworth, 1973), pp. 51–91.

12. Warren, "On the Moral and Legal Status of Abortion," p. 117.

13. Warren, "On the Moral and Legal Status of Abortion," p. 112.

14. Warren, "On the Moral and Legal Status of Abortion," pp. 115–116.

15. Tooley, "A Defense of Abortion and Infanticide," pp. 79–89.

16. See L. W. Sumner, *Abortion and Moral Theory* (Princeton, NJ: Princeton University Press, 1981), pp. 99–106.

17. See Philip E. Devine, *The Ethics of Homicide* (Ithaca, NY: Cornell University Press, 1978), p. 99.

18. The first version of the moderate position sketched here is based on elements from two essays, both in Feinberg, *The Problem of Abortion*. They are Judith Jarvis Thomson, "A Defense of Abortion," pp. 173–187, and Jane English, "Abortion and the Concept of a Person," pp. 151–160.

19. See especially Thomson, "A Defense of Abortion," pp. 180–182. The reason for the qualification "unjustly" is to allow for cases such as killing in self-defense.

20. See Tom L. Beauchamp and James F. Childress, *Principles of Biomedical Ethics*, 4th ed. (New York: Oxford University Press, 1994), pp. 192, 266–267.

21. For another case that illustrates this same point about the law in the United States, see "Mrs. X and the Bone Marrow Transplant," in Carol Levine (ed.), *Cases in Bioethics* (New York: St. Martin's Press, 1989), pp. 180–185.

22. Edward A. Langerak, "Abortion: Listening to the Middle," in John Arras and Nancy Rhoden (eds.), *Ethical Issues in Modern Medicine*, 3d ed. (Mountain View, CA: Mayfield, 1989), pp. 286–292.

23. Sumner, *Abortion and Moral Theory*, especially Chapter 4.

24. For the full argument, see Sumner, *Abortion and Moral Theory*, pp. 146–154.

CHAPTER 6

Experimentation
and the Use
of Human Subjects

THROUGHOUT THIS BOOK we have seen that individual autonomy and well-being are two basic values that ought to be respected and promoted. As we learned in previous chapters, these values can conflict. Telling competent patients the truth respects their autonomy but may occasionally adversely affect their well-being. Breaching the confidence of a competent patient or treating that patient without fully informed consent may promote well-being but at the expense of autonomy. And utilitarian considerations, understood in terms of the well-being of the whole, are important too. In this chapter, we will be discussing medical research and the use of human beings as experimental subjects. As we shall see, this topic, too, reveals a conflict between basic values.

Health care professionals, qua health care professionals, sometimes play two different roles. On the one hand, they are therapists. As therapists, they have an obligation to promote the health and well-being of their patients. On the other hand, some health care professionals are involved in research as well. As scientists, they are seeking to advance the growth of knowledge. That many people in the field of medicine play each of these roles is clear; that doing so can lead to moral problems may be less clear. Occupying these two different roles can lead to a problem of conflicting loyalties. What one ought to do as a researcher may conflict with what one ought to do as a therapist. Doing what will best promote advances in medical knowledge may require doing things that are in conflict with therapists' obligations.

The goal of research is the acquisition of generalizable knowledge. In the context of medical research, sometimes the promotion of that goal may require that subjects be placed at risk. Thus, the utilitarian end conflicts with the well-being of individuals. On other occasions, the promotion of that end may require that subjects be deceived, which is contrary to autonomy. These are the conflicts that we shall discuss, beginning with the basic framework.

THE FRAMEWORK

In looking at medical experiments, the most basic question we might ask is "Who are the subjects?" Here we shall be concerned with research involving human subjects. We would be remiss, however, not to mention that most medical research involves nonhuman animals. And there are many important ethical questions to ask about this research. Are the animals harmed by their participation in the experiments? Do the experiments really produce benefits for people? Is any other way possible to achieve the benefits? And even if benefits are produced and there is no other way to do so, does that justify inflicting harm on animals? These are important questions. But our focus will be on research involving human subjects.

As difficult as the issues about the use of animals are, if all medical research involved only animals as subjects, matters would be simpler. But in medicine, experimenting on human subjects is necessary for several reasons. First, different drugs and treatments sometimes have different effects on different species. As a result, when anything new is tried for the first time on humans, it is experimental. Also, some medical problems are unique to human beings. If any progress is to be made on the treatment of these problems, human beings must be used as subjects.

In examining medical experiments that use human subjects, the most fundamental question concerns whether the research is therapeutic or nontherapeutic. *Therapeutic research*, like all research, is concerned with the acquisition of generalizable knowledge. But therapeutic research is expected to benefit the patient-subjects directly. It may involve testing a new drug, treatment, or diagnostic procedure with the expectation that the subjects will benefit. Such research is designed to benefit the subjects by their very participation. By contrast, *nontherapeutic research* involves the acquisition of generalizable knowledge and new information that one hopes will be helpful to future patients. No direct medical benefits are expected for the subjects; if there are any medical benefits for the subjects, they are unexpected side effects.

Another crucial question is whether the subject is competent. In this context, the issue is whether the subject is qualified to decide for herself to participate in the experiment. Among many other things, competence requires an ability to assess the benefits and risks of participation. When a potential subject is not competent, a legal guardian must make the decision.

If the subject is competent, we must then ask whether she has consented to participate in the experiment. As in Chapter 3, here "consent" means more than just saying yes. Consent is genuine only if it is freely given and fully informed. Consent is freely given if no pressure or coercion is exerted on the subjects and if the subjects did not agree under duress. For consent to be fully informed, the subjects must understand the purpose of the experiments and the risks and benefits likely to result from their participation.

Another important issue concerns whether risks are involved to those who participate in the research. Risks might entail either bodily or emotional harm. As with informed consent to treatment, decisions must be made about what risks to inform subjects about, for some risks are very unlikely to occur. Based on these distinctions, many possibilities emerge. With research that is therapeutic, we can highlight two possibilities: when the subjects have consented and when they have not consented. Therapeutic research with the consent of the subjects is just a special case of patients consenting to treatment. No moral problems need arise here. Therapeutic research without the consent of the subjects is a special case of treatment without consent, and that topic was addressed in detail in Chapter 3. So here we shall confine our discussion to nontherapeutic research.

When research is nontherapeutic, we have four interesting possibilities: the subjects have consented and there are no risks; the subjects have consented and there are risks; the subjects have not consented and there are no risks; and the subjects have not consented and there are risks. The first of these four seems morally unproblematic; when the subjects' consent is freely given and fully informed and there are no serious risks, no serious moral problem is apparent. The other three possibilities do raise moral issues. If the subjects have consented but there are significant risks involved, we may wonder whether the experiment should be allowed. This, among other things, raises questions of paternalism. If the subjects have not consented but there is no risk to them, the experiment will compromise their autonomy. And if the subjects have not given genuine consent and there are risks involved, both their autonomy and well-being are compromised. Later in this chapter we shall look at examples of each of these three possibilities.

If the subjects are not competent and the research is nontherapeutic, two questions arise. First, has the legal guardian given genuine consent? Second, are there any risks to the subjects by their participation? Again, this situation gives rise to four possibilities. We shall later discuss some of these as they apply to the use of children as experimental subjects.

Before looking at examples, however, we shall briefly consider what some of the codes of ethics say about experimentation.

CODES OF ETHICS AND EXPERIMENTATION

Several professional codes of ethics address issues involving the use of human subjects. Here we shall discuss the Nuremberg Code, the Declaration of Helsinki, and the American Medical Association Ethical Guidelines for Clinical Investigation. (Each is reprinted in the Appendix.)

The Nuremberg Code

Published in 1948, the Nuremberg Code was written in response to Nazi atrocities, especially those involving the use of human beings as experimental subjects. This code sometimes seems extreme, but understanding its historical roots explains its intent.

The first article of the Nuremberg Code states, "The voluntary consent of the human subject is *absolutely* essential." And lest this statement be misinterpreted, its meaning is spelled out in detail. Persons being used as research subjects must have the legal capacity to give consent. Subjects must be capable of exercising free power of choice, without any element of force, fraud, deceit, duress, constraint, or coercion. Subjects must have a sufficient knowledge of the nature of the experiment so that they can make an informed decision about participation. Researchers must explain the nature, purpose, and duration of the experiment to the subjects. The subjects must be made aware of all inconveniences, hazards, and possible adverse effects on their health that might reasonably be expected to result from their participation in the experiment. Those who initiate, direct, and engage in the experiment are responsible for ascertaining the quality of the consent.

Several points in the Nuremberg Code are worth highlighting. First, the requirement for voluntary consent is absolute; the code allows for no exceptions. Second, because subjects must have the legal capacity to give consent, it follows that children may never be used as subjects, though the code does not explicitly say this. Third, the code requires that subjects be informed as to the nature and purposes of the experiment and of any possible risks involved. This is the requirement of informed consent. Finally, this code, unlike others, makes no distinction between therapeutic and nontherapeutic experiments.

The Declaration of Helsinki

The Declaration of Helsinki was adopted by the Eighteenth World Medical Assembly in 1964 in Helsinki, Finland, and revised by the Twenty-Ninth World Medical Assembly in 1975 in Tokyo, Japan. The Declaration of Helsinki emphasizes the distinction between therapeutic and nontherapeutic experiments. The reason for emphasizing this distinction, presumably, is that researchers should be given more moral leeway if a research project is therapeutic. The declaration has distinct guidelines for the two types of experiments.

Concerning therapeutic research, the following are some of the main points made in the Declaration of Helsinki. First, in treating patients, physicians must be free to use new unproven therapeutic measures if in their judgment doing so offers hope of saving life, restoring health, or alleviating suffering. Second, if possible, the physician should obtain the patient's freely given and fully informed consent. However, if the physician considers it essential not to obtain informed consent, then the reasons for this should be stated in the experimental protocol and assessed by an independent committee. This measure presumably allows for paternalism in certain cases because the physician's reasons for not seeking informed consent will likely refer to the well-being of the patient-subject. If the patient is legally incompetent, then consent should be obtained from the legal guardian. Third, physicians may combine clinical research with professional care only to the extent that the clinical research is justified by its expected therapeutic value for the subjects. In other words, physicians may use their patients as experimental subjects only if it is reasonable to expect that there will be direct medical benefits for those patient-subjects. The authors of this code were sensitive to the potential difficulties involved when physicians use their own patients as subjects in an experiment, and so they required that it be expected that the subjects will benefit medically from participation. The implication is that health care professionals may not use their own patients as subjects in a nontherapeutic experiment. The authors were especially concerned about this point because patients may feel pressured to participate; they may feel that their care will be compromised if they do not agree to be a subject. As a result, the consent given may be compromised.

Concerning nontherapeutic experimentation, the following are among the declaration's guidelines. (Some of these points apply to therapeutic research as well.) First, the nature and purpose of the experiment and the potential risks of participation must be explained to the subjects by the physician-researcher. Second, at all times during the experiment physicians must protect the life and health of the subjects. If the life or well-being of a subject is in danger, the experiment should be stopped. Third, the freely given, fully informed consent of subjects must be obtained. If the subject is legally incompetent, the consent of the legal guardian must be procured. Fourth, it is preferable that consent be obtained in writing. Fifth, it must be made clear to the subjects or guardians that they are free to withdraw from the experiment at any time. Sixth, any research involving human subjects should be formulated in an experimental protocol and examined by an independent committee. Such committees are called institutional review boards (IRBs), and in the United States federally funded institutions doing research on human subjects must have an IRB.

We might note briefly some differences between the Declaration of Helsinki and the Nuremberg Code. First, the declaration does make a distinction between therapeutic and nontherapeutic research. Second, the declaration suggests that it is appropriate to grant physician-researchers more liberties regarding the former than the latter. In particular, in some cases therapeutic research may be initiated without the patient's consent. Finally, unlike the Nuremberg Code, the Declaration of Helsinki explicitly allows the use of incompetents in nontherapeutic research if the consent of the legal guardian is obtained.

American Medical Association Ethical
Guidelines for Clinical Investigation

In 1966, the American Medical Association Ethical Guidelines for Clinical Investigation were issued. Like the Declaration of Helsinki, these guidelines distinguish explicitly between "clinical investigation primarily for treatment" and "clinical investigation primarily for the accumulation of scientific knowledge." Again, restrictions on the use of human subjects differ in these two cases.

Concerning therapeutic experimentation, the AMA guidelines include the following provisions. First, normally physicians should obtain consent from patients when using investigational drugs or experimental procedures. Physicians should provide a reasonable explanation of the nature of the drug or procedure to be used and should explain the possible risks and expected therapeutic benefits. However, if the physician judges that disclosure of such information would likely affect the health of the patient adversely or would be detrimental to the patient's best interests, such information may be withheld. This approach is paternalistic, strongly so if the patient is competent. Second, if emergency treatment is necessary, the patient is incapable of giving consent, and no one is available who has the authority to speak for the patient, consent may be assumed. As with the more general topic of treatment without consent, this clause endorses only weak paternalism.

Concerning investigation that is primarily for the accumulation of scientific knowledge, the AMA guidelines are very similar to the recommendations of the Declaration of Helsinki. The one noteworthy difference, however, concerns the use of minors and mentally incompetent adults in nontherapeutic experiments. The Declaration of Helsinki merely requires that the informed consent of the legal guardian be obtained. The AMA guidelines also require that the freely given and fully informed consent of the legal guardian be obtained before a minor or mentally incompetent person may be used as a subject in a nontherapeutic experiment. But the guidelines also require the satisfaction of a second condition. "The nature of the investigation is such that mentally competent adults would not be suitable subjects." A competent adult will not be a suitable subject if the investigation is directed specifically at a medical problem that only children experience or that afflicts only mentally retarded persons. In either of these cases, to make progress on the problem in question, children or mentally disabled persons must be used as subjects.

In summary, then, the Nuremberg Code allows no experimentation without the consent of the subject-patient; the Declaration of Helsinki and the AMA guidelines permit therapeutic experiments without consent only if the physician judges that seeking consent is inadvisable or when the patient cannot consent. Concerning the use of children or mental incompetents as subjects, the Nuremberg Code forbids it; the Declaration of Helsinki allows it if the legal guardian has consented; and the AMA guidelines permit it only if the guardian has consented and a competent adult could not serve as a suitable subject in the experiment. In all cases, the Nuremberg Code is understandably the most restrictive. Regarding the use of incompetents as subjects, the AMA guidelines are more permissive than the Nuremberg Code, which forbids their use, but less permissive than the Declaration of Helsinki, which requires only the guardian's consent.

NONTHERAPEUTIC EXPERIMENTS:
THE MORAL ISSUES

As indicated, when an experiment is nontherapeutic and the subjects are competent, four types of cases must be discussed: the subjects have consented and there is no risk; the subjects have consented and there is risk; the subjects have not consented and there is no risk; and the subjects have not consented and there is risk. These four types of situations will be discussed, and then case studies illustrating each of the last three will be presented.

In type 1 cases, in which the subjects are competent, have given consent, and face no risks, no moral problems are evident. This is simply a case of people choosing to volunteer, either for altruistic or monetary reasons. In such situations, all that needs to be done is ensure that the subjects' consent was freely given and fully informed. Ensuring this may not be easy. In the past, prisoners, students, and very poor persons were the most frequent experimental subjects, and many doubted that their consent was freely given. The issue here is whether those in economic dire straits can freely consent to participate in an experiment in which they are paid. Some are also skeptical that subjects are adequately informed. They claim that scientific complexities render *informed* consent virtually impossible.[1] A full discussion of these issues is not possible here. Instead, simply note that for cases of this first sort, the main issue is whether the subjects' consent was freely given and fully informed.

In type 2 cases, in which the subjects are competent, have given consent, but the experiment involves risk to the subjects, the issue is whether such experiments may be prohibited to prevent the potential harm. The argument in favor of permitting such research protocols appeals to the right of autonomy of the subjects. As long as their consent is genuine, they alone should decide the appropriateness of participating.

What grounds are there for opposing experiments of type 2? One obvious basis for opposition is strong paternalism. Here one might propose prohibiting such experiments for the purpose of preventing harm to the subjects. Because the subjects have given genuine consent, preventing their participation for their own good is strongly paternalistic. But this is not the only basis for opposing such research. A second possibility appeals to the adverse effects on the medical profession as a whole. The principal goal of health care professionals is to promote their patients' health and well-being. Indeed, health care practitioners often chide patients who engage in unhealthy behavior, such as smoking and eating a poor diet. For members of this same profession to participate in activities in which people are knowingly subjecting themselves to risk seems odd. Such a practice may lead to serious mistrust and damage the reputation of the profession. If so, we have a nonpaternalistic reason to oppose experiments of type 2. Note, however, this point. If the state, through the arm of the law, were to prohibit experiments of this sort, presumably its basis would be paternalistic. The nonpaternalistic basis for opposing these experiments would presumably come from the medical professions themselves; the limitation would be self-imposed. And perhaps this nonpaternalistic reason for opposing such research does not apply to professions that do not mete out health care and do not depend greatly on public trust—for example, experimental psychologists.

The third possibility involves nontherapeutic research in which there is no risk to the subjects, but the subjects did not consent. Recall that "consent" means more than saying yes. In typical cases of this type, the subjects have agreed to participate, but their consent is compromised. The consent is either not freely given or not fully informed, as our case studies will show. The argument in support of permitting such research is utilitarian, appealing to the overall good that will result from it. The utilitarian argument says that such experiments should be permitted if the following three conditions are satisfied: (1) there is no risk to the subjects; (2) considerable benefits can result from such experiments, ultimately leading to improvements for future patients; and (3) these benefits cannot be obtained if the subjects' consent is required. Condition 3 might be true either because nobody would consent if asked or because obtaining consent would ruin the experiment. Again, case studies will illustrate this point.

The main reason for opposing experiments of type 3 is that they violate the subjects' right to self-determination. Even if the subjects are not harmed or placed at risk, they are still being manipulated. And such manipulation interferes with the subjects' autonomy. Note that in discussing previous issues we considered cases where it may be appropriate to act against the autonomy of the patient. In the Tarasoff case (Chapter 2), for example, many held that the psychologist should have breached confidence for the good of the whole. But there is a significant difference between that case and experiments of type 3. In the Tarasoff case, if Poddar's confidence is breached, it is to prevent him from harming another innocent person. But in type 3 experiments, if we use subjects without their full consent, we are in effect forcing them to benefit others, which seems like a more serious infringement of liberty. Still, it should be emphasized that experiments of type 3 present us with a difficult issue. For if it is really true that certain important benefits can be obtained only if we engage in such research, then we must choose between an important utilitarian goal and the autonomy of individual subjects.

The fourth possibility concerns nontherapeutic research in which the subjects did not consent and there is risk involved. Again, the subjects may have agreed to participate; but something, typically deception, undermined the genuineness of their consent. Again, the argument in support of such research is utilitarian, appealing to the future good to be obtained. According to the utilitarian argument, such experiments should be permitted if two conditions are satisfied: (1) the benefits likely to accrue for others—cures for future patients—outweigh the harm that will be done to the subjects; and (2) these benefits cannot be obtained if the subjects' consent is required. Again, condition 2 is true in certain cases because subjects probably would not agree to participate if they were fully informed; it is also possible that their consent would ruin the experiment.

The reasons for opposing experiments of type 4 are clear: they compromise both the subjects' autonomy and well-being. Because informed consent is not obtained, the subjects' right to self-determination is violated. And because risk is involved, subjects are unwittingly putting themselves in a position to be harmed.

It should be emphasized that the three difficult cases—2, 3, and 4—involve conflicts among the basic values that have been stressed in this book. The good of the whole is important, and that good is promoted by promising research. But in certain cases that good can be achieved only by compromising the autonomy or well-being of experimental subjects. In those cases, we face decisions where we lose something either way.

CASE STUDIES

Having described the various sorts of nontherapeutic experiments, we shall now look at particular cases illustrating types 2, 3, and 4.

Cases of Type 2

One example of an experiment of this sort is described by Robert M. Veatch,[2] presented here in a modified form. This 1964 protocol was designed to study the effects of LSD on the individual's personality. Some prospective subjects knew little or nothing about LSD, and so whether they could give informed consent is doubtful. But consider only those prospective subjects who knew a considerable amount about LSD. (Those who had previous experience with LSD were disqualified.) At the outset, subjects were given a battery of personality tests. During a one-hour interview, they were told that they might or might not receive LSD. Questions pertaining to the safety of LSD were answered during the interview, but no mention was made of possibility of personality changes for fear that this would ruin the experiment. Some subjects received LSD, and some received an amphetamine. The experiment was double-blind; that is, neither researchers nor subjects knew who was being given what drug. On the days that drugs were administered, subjects were attended to all day for their safety.

The fact that subjects were not told about possible personality changes obviously creates doubts that their consent was adequately informed, though it may be true that informing them of this possibility would have distorted the results. But put that aside for now, and focus instead on the risks involved in this study. Can experiments that impose great risks on the subjects if those subjects' consent is freely given and fully informed be justified? It is worth recalling that if the state were to ban such experiments, such a prohibition would be an instance of strong paternalism. But the medical profession, policing itself, might recommend against such studies on grounds that it is wrong for health care professionals to encourage people to engage in risky behavior and doing so may damage significantly the reputation of the profession. If such experiments are prohibited absolutely, however, society will be depriving itself of much knowledge, knowledge that may be quite useful. A second example illustrates this.

This case was described recently by Terrence F. Ackerman and Carson Strong.[3] The protocol in question is designed to determine the advantages of buffered over regular aspirin in providing protection to stomach linings. Aspirin can exacerbate many problems, including peptic ulcers and stomach distress. The objective of this study is to determine whether aspirin with buffering ingredients will significantly decrease the impact of acid on the stomach lining. Only healthy, competent adult subjects were to be used. Four medications were to be compared, including two forms of buffered aspirin. Each subject would take one drug for three days, and then take the second, third, and fourth drugs in subsequent three-day trial periods. The effects of each drug on the stomach lining were to be ascertained by inspection of the lining, employing a procedure known as endoscopy. During each three-day trial period, subjects would undergo three endoscopies. Trial periods would be separated by a seven-day break. As a result, twelve endoscopies would be performed on each subject over a period of thirty-three days. Endoscopy involves the passage of a flexible tube through the mouth and into the gastrointestinal tract. Approximately one hour before the procedure, subjects will be given a sedative but not anesthetized. Immediately before the procedure a modest amount of topical anesthesia will be applied. The amount of pain and discomfort associated with the procedure varies from subject to subject. Most persons gag for a brief period. When air is pumped into the stomach, subjects will feel bloated. Discomfort, rather than actual risk, is the principal side effect.

Performing twelve nontherapeutic endoscopies over a period of approximately a month is troubling. Some might even wonder how an informed person could agree to undergo these procedures. Still, the knowledge sought in this study was potentially quite useful. Is it appropriate to allow informed subjects to partake in such a study? One difference between this and the LSD study concerns the harm that might befall the subjects. In the LSD experiment, the risks may be quite great. In the latter study, however, some might even deny that there are serious risks. Those who make such a denial, presumably, distinguish between discomforts and risks and say that only discomfort is involved with the nontherapeutic endoscopy. The distinction is legitimate; what is not clear is whether we should be cavalier about allowing subjects to put themselves in a position of experiencing repeated discomforts.

Cases of Type 3

One well-known example of a nontherapeutic experiment involving no risks to the subjects but in which the consent of the subjects is compromised is the case of the Jewish Chronic Disease Hospital. This study will be described in detail here.

The case at the Jewish Chronic Disease Hospital occurred in 1963 and drew a lot of publicity in 1964.[4] It involved two doctors, Emanuel Mandel, medical director of the Chronic Disease Hospital, and Chester Southam, the person directing the research in question. Southam was doing research in cancer immunology and was involved in a project in which cultured cancer cells were being injected into hospitalized patients. His work at the Chronic Disease Hospital involved twenty-two seriously ill and debilitated patients who served as subjects. Within the scientific community, Southam's research on cancer immunology was thought to be important.

Upon receiving Mandel's approval, Southam conducted one phase of his research on twenty-two patients in the Chronic Disease Hospital. The goal was to determine the speed with which the injected cancer cells were rejected by the body. Earlier phases of Southam's research demonstrated that healthy persons reject cancer cells in four to six weeks, but persons with advanced cancer take a longer time to reject such cells, sometimes up to three months. Southam wanted to explain this slower rate of rejection. The obvious hypothesis was that the slower rate of rejection in cancer patients was attributable to the fact that they had cancer. But another hypothesis seemed equally plausible: the slower rate of rejection was due to the general debility that accompanies any chronic illness. To confirm the first hypothesis, Southam needed to conduct an experiment on patients with chronic but nonmalignant illnesses. Where better to find such subjects than the Jewish Chronic Disease Hospital.

Having secured an agreement from Mandel to collaborate on this project, they selected twenty-two patients from the institution. Three had cancer and served as controls; the other nineteen had chronic, nonmalignant illnesses. Each of the patient-subjects was asked to consent to an injection that was described as a test to discover resistance or immunity to disease. They were told, correctly, that a lump would form and that in a few weeks it would go away. They were not told that this procedure was unrelated to their own condition, nor were they told that the substance to be injected was cancer cells. According to the record, all of the subjects agreed to the injection, and none suffered any ill effects.

When knowledge of this experiment became public, Southam and Mandel were widely criticized. The adverse publicity prompted the Division of Professional Conduct of the State of New York to address the case. The Regents of the University of the State of New York had to investigate because they were responsible for licensing the medical profession. The charges against the two physicians were "unprofessional conduct" and "fraud and deceit in the practice of medicine." The critics charged that they took advantage of chronically ill patients.

Southam and Mandel offered a spirited defense of the research. The first point they made was that the experiments involved no harm or risk to the subjects. They were correct in asserting this, but critics did not claim that harm to the subjects was the basis for objecting to the experiments. Second, Southam and Mandel argued that the consent of the patient-subjects had been obtained. No one disputed that the subjects agreed to participate; what was at issue was the quality of their consent. Critics asked why the subjects were not fully informed about the nature of the procedure. In particular, why were they not told that they were being injected with cancer cells? The researchers claimed that the word *cancer* was not used because that word was not pertinent to the experience that the subjects would have. Moreover, it has emotional disvalue. Many prospective subjects would experience irrational fear upon hearing that cancer cells would be injected into their bodies. Southam and Mandel were, in effect, offering the classical utilitarian argument for the research: significant benefits could come from this experiment, no harm would come to the subjects, and these benefits could not be achieved if the subjects' fully informed consent were required.

As a third point, Southam and Mandel claimed that the subjects benefited from their participation in the experiment. Although sounding odd initially, their contention was that the patient-subjects received more attention, which improved their care. Fourth, lawyers for these physicians argued that at the time of their actions there were no unequivocal professional standards that they violated. As a result, if they were found guilty and punished, it would be a case of *ex post facto* legislation. Finally, the lawyers claimed that many other members of the medical profession followed the practices and procedures used by Southam and Mandel. If the conduct is widespread within the profession, it cannot be "unprofessional," they reasoned.

In spite of this defense, the doctors lost. Their penalty, however, was light; their licenses were suspended for one year, but the execution of the sentence was stayed. As a result, they were put on probation for one year and permitted to continue the practice of medicine.

The principal points made against Southam and Mandel's research protocol were important. First, some claimed that this experiment was nontherapeutic. Southam and Mandel maintained that their subjects stood to benefit because they would receive closer attention and care. Critics did not deny this but argued that such benefits were incidental and not central to the purpose of the experiment. The existence of side benefits does not make research therapeutic; an experiment must have as its principal aim the benefit of the patient-subjects to be therapeutic. This point is important because if the broader notion of "therapeutic" were accepted, practically every experiment would be therapeutic, and the distinction would be lost.

Second, though the subjects did agree to participate in the experiment, their consent was not genuine; they were not given the information needed for their consent to be fully informed. Southam and Mandel claimed that the information that they withheld from the subjects was not needed to make a rational decision about participation. The counter, however, was that it is the subjects who have the right to decide what factors are relevant to their decision, regardless of whether anyone else thinks those factors are important. Subjects have a right to know all material facts and may refuse to participate for any reason whatsoever. Even if the experiment will benefit some and harm no one, fully informed consent is necessary. The criticism rejects the utilitarian argument and affirms the importance of self-determination. The effect here is to claim that the subjects were manipulated by deliberate nondisclosure of material facts. This point is important, but there is a gap. It is implausible to think that researchers can explain *every* fact about an experiment to the subjects. And it is hard to see how researchers can know what any particular subject might consider relevant.[5] Perhaps what is needed here is something like the "reasonable person" standard discussed in connection with informed consent to treatment in Chapter 3.

Finally, critics questioned the quality of the subjects' consent, independent of the omitted information. In some cases, they felt that the competence of the subjects was questionable. But they were also concerned that the subjects were weak and perhaps therefore consent was given under duress. Another concern was this: to the extent that Mandel was involved in this research and the recruitment of subjects, patients may feel, perhaps unjustifiably, that their care would be compromised if they refused to participate. This point reminds us of the wisdom of the Declaration of Helsinki's requirement that physicians not use their own patients as subjects in nontherapeutic research.

Another interesting example of a type 3 case was described recently by Ackerman and Strong.[6] This case involves research on alcoholism. As many as 10 percent of American men and 5 percent of American women are estimated to be alcoholics. Alcoholism leads, directly or indirectly, to many deaths and numerous other problems. Identifying alcoholics is therefore quite important. But physicians may fail to diagnose accurately at least half of their patients who are alcoholics. There are, of course, many reasons for this, including the proclivity of alcoholics to hide or deny their symptoms. Therefore, tests to better enable physicians to screen patients for alcohol dependence would be desirable.

In the case Ackerman and Strong discuss, a research protocol was proposed that would help physicians identify persons dependent on alcohol. One aspect of the protocol involved an interview in which subjects would be asked various questions about their medical histories, in particular about the use of alcohol. Another aspect involved testing the blood for various chemical substances. After securing consent, a nurse would conduct the interview and draw the blood. The problem, however, concerned informed consent. To receive accurate answers to the interview questions, the researchers believed that they could not fully explain the purpose of the study to the subjects because prospective subjects who did abuse alcohol would likely either give false answers to avoid detection or decline to participate. So the researchers needed to withhold information about the purpose of the experiment to get accurate information from the subjects and produce useful results.

Clearly this experiment is nontherapeutic and has the potential to produce important information that will benefit many. And the researchers' claim that fully informed consent would distort the results seems plausible. So we have here an example where we are forced to choose between the utilitarian good for all of society and the rights of individual subjects.

A Case of Type 4

Probably the most infamous study in the United States is the Tuskegee Syphilis Experiment.[7] In 1929, the syphilis rate in Macon County, Alabama, was 40 percent, the highest in the nation. Under the auspices of the U.S. Public Health Service, a program was set up to detect and treat blacks with syphilis in Macon County. At the time, mercury ointment was the available treatment. In 1932, however, funds ran out and the program was turned into a nontherapeutic study lasting for four decades. The chief physician in charge saw this as an "unparalleled opportunity" to observe the effects of untreated syphilis in blacks.

Approximately 400 black men with late-stage syphilis were to be observed but not treated. This study was developed in part because physicians believed that long-term syphilis might not be as bad as antisyphilis crusaders had claimed. The idea was to study the progression of untreated syphilis and develop the natural history of that disease. Syphilis becomes latent for many years and is difficult to diagnose during that stage. It gradually affects the nervous and circulatory systems.

The men being observed in this study did not know that they had syphilis; doctors told them that they were being treated for "bad blood." They were given free transportation to the clinic and a meal to induce them to participate. They were observed quite irregularly because funding for the study was uneven, which made their observations less reliable. By 1933 physicians had discovered a number of cases of cardiovascular syphilis, which adversely affects the spinal cord. Physicians tricked these patients into coming for painful spinal taps by sending them a letter inviting them to come for "a special treatment." This was necessary to observe how far the syphilis had progressed. After World War II, penicillin was available as a treatment for syphilis, but the men in this study never received it. In fact, in the late 1960s the Macon County Medical Society was given a list of all individuals in the study and agreed not to give them antibiotics for any condition.

Curiously, this study was not entirely secret. It was described in a 1936 article in the prestigious *Journal of the American Medical Association*.[8] It was apparently little noticed, or people simply were not outraged. But in 1966, Peter Buxtun, a venereal disease investigator, learned of the study and criticized officials of the U.S. Public Health Service for permitting its continuation. He got nowhere, however. In 1972, he told an Associated Press reporter about the study. Jean Heller was assigned to investigate, and on July 26, 1972, the story ran in newspapers around the country. This publicity led to the termination of the study. A class action suit was settled out of court in 1974. Men still living received approximately $37,000; heirs of the deceased received $15,000.

Another example of a type 4 case has recently been brought to the public's attention. Between 1944 and 1974, the U.S. government sponsored a variety of experiments in which individuals were deliberately exposed to radiation without their knowledge. In January 1994, President Bill Clinton appointed an advisory committee that studied hundreds of documents from various governmental agencies. Its final report documented many shocking experiments, including feeding radioactive cereal to mentally disabled teenagers, irradiating prisoners' testicles, and injecting plutonium into hospital patients.[9] Known collectively as "the human radiation experiments," these studies were conducted during the Cold War, presumably to acquire knowledge that might advance efforts being made at the time against the former Soviet Union.

These are horrible episodes in our history. They are also bad examples of type 4 cases because it is hard to see here how the utilitarian argument in defense of such experiments applies; surely the possible benefits that might have come from them could not outweigh the harm done to the subjects. In this respect, we need better examples.

MUST CONSENT ALWAYS BE OBTAINED?

Cases of type 3 and 4 raise the issue of whether it is ever morally permissible to engage in a nontherapeutic research protocol without the subjects' fully informed consent. This is important and challenging because there may be utilitarian gains that are virtually unachievable if informed consent is required. It will be very difficult to justify type 4 cases because of the risks imposed on the subjects. If there is any hope, it lies in cases of type 3.

Robert Veatch discusses an interesting case of this sort.[10] Several researchers were involved in testing psychoactive drugs. In doing so, they always had to use a control group to whom a placebo was given. These scientists explained the risks involved and obtained the subjects' consent. One thing, however, they could not explain. Some of the subjects would be receiving medication known to be ineffective. If the subjects were told this, researchers believed that the experiment would be ruined. But disagreement arose among the researchers. Some wanted to tell all subjects that some of them would be receiving placebos; others felt that this would cause some of the subjects to report their perceptions inaccurately and thus compromise the experiment. After discussion, the doctors decided to do a study to determine the effects of telling subjects that they have a chance of receiving a placebo. One group would be told that each of them had one chance in four of receiving a placebo. This information would not be given to the other group, though in fact each of them too had a one in four chance of receiving a placebo. Clearly, this is a nontherapeutic experiment. It is also plausible to say that the possible benefits of this study are significant. For if it were to turn out that telling subjects that they have a chance of receiving a placebo did not affect the results of the experiment, all future researchers could obtain fully informed consent when conducting similar experiments. Yet in this particular experiment, consent cannot be obtained because the goal is to determine whether informing subjects makes any difference.

This experiment reveals a difficult choice: in some cases, either we must use human beings as experimental subjects without their fully informed consent, or there is certain knowledge that we may never justifiably pursue. Neither of these choices seems acceptable. It is undesirable to place the pursuit of certain knowledge out of reach. But we are appropriately reticent about using people as subjects without their informed consent. Veatch suggests avoiding this dilemma by invoking the notion of "implied consent." "The implied consent of the real subjects may reasonably be assumed if, and only if, there is good evidence that a reasonable person would consent if he had been adequately informed."[11]

How do we determine whether a reasonable person would consent to participate in a given study? Veatch suggests that a mock subject group be selected from the same population as the real subjects. The nature, purpose, and possible risks of the experiment should be explained to this mock group, and then they should be asked whether they would consent to be subjects in such an experiment. If an overwhelming majority say that they would consent, then researchers can reasonably assume that the real subjects would consent too. This approach would allow society to pursue nontherapeutic experiments that are important and are such that actual consent would ruin the experiment.

Veatch's proposal is thought-provoking. Its appeal lies in the fact that it seems to provide a way of pursuing certain appropriate utilitarian goals without ignoring completely self-determination. We conclude here with two brief remarks. First, if the purpose of requiring consent is to respect people's right to self-determination, then Veatch's proposal does not succeed. The consent of hypothetical subjects may indicate that the actual subjects' well-being will not be threatened, but that is different from respecting autonomy. Second, asking people whether they *would* consent under certain circumstances may not produce the same answers as asking them if they *do* consent. It may be much easier to give hypothetical consent.

RANDOM CLINICAL TRIALS

For new drugs, treatments, and diagnostic procedures to be made available to patients as part of routine medicine, they must be adequately tested to determine their efficacy. Testing drugs goes through various stages. A *phase I* trial attempts merely to establish the safety of an agent, for example, to determine its levels of toxicity. A *phase II* trial looks for promise of efficacy by examining the effects of the drug on a small number of subjects who are likely to benefit from it. A *phase III* trial seeks definitive evidence of efficacy by comparing the experimental agent with currently used therapies or with a placebo. At this stage the drug is administered to a large number of patients by many different clinical investigators. Such trials typically take place at teaching hospitals or large public institutions. If the results are successful, the drug will likely be licensed for general use. At this third stage, random clinical trials are typically used; they are also used to test diagnostic procedures and new treatments.

The purpose of a random clinical trial (RCT) is to determine the effectiveness of a treatment, often in comparison with some other treatment.[12] There must be at least two groups of subjects: one receiving the experimental treatment and the control group. The control group will receive either the standard treatment, if any is available, or a placebo, something believed to have no biological effect. The idea is to determine whether the experimental treatment is better than the standard treatment or better than a mere placebo. The reason for the latter is that people who are ill and who believe that a physician can help them typically show improvement when a physician does something merely because of that belief. When no standard treatment is available, a control group receiving a placebo is necessary to determine whether improvements are due to biological effects or placebo effects. In addition, mere improvement does not prove the effectiveness of a treatment, for an illness may have simply run its course. Again, the control group receiving a placebo enables researchers to determine this. An RCT attempts to construct two groups that are alike in all relevant respects except that one receives the experimental treatment and the other is the control group.

Assignment to the experimental group or the control group is done randomly. The goal is to distribute randomly the many possible influencing factors so that any difference in outcome can be attributed to a difference in the treatment. Random assignment is also necessary to eliminate bias in the selection of treatment. For researchers might subconsciously assign less ill patients to the experimental group, thus resulting in a distorted view of the treatment's efficacy.

Often RCTs are double-blind, which means that neither the researchers nor the patient-subjects know who is receiving the experimental treatment and who is in the control group. The purpose of this approach is to eliminate bias. Investigators want their tests to be successful and so may "perceive" a patient as "improved"; patients want to get better and so may "feel" better. So, either of these participants may have distorted views of the results if they know who is receiving the experimental treatment. When an RCT is double-blind, treatment assignments are coded, and the "blinders" are removed later. Not all RCTs are double-blind. Some may be single-blind, where only the researchers know who is receiving what, and some may not be blind at all because it is not possible. Examples of the latter are (1) comparing a lumpectomy, a lumpectomy plus radiation, and a simple mastectomy as treatments for breast cancer and (2) comparing amputation alone with amputation plus chemotherapy for certain types of cancer. In these two cases, it is understandably much more difficult to get patients to agree to a random assignment of treatment.

An RCT must be constructed so that the result is statistically significant. Enough patients must be given the experimental treatment to ensure that the results are due to the treatment and not mere chance. If you tossed a coin three times, and it came up heads each time, you would not have grounds for concluding that the coin was somehow rigged. But if you tossed the coin twenty-five times and it came up heads each time, matters would be different. In RCTs, matters are more complicated, but there must be enough trials to produce significant results. Researchers consult with statisticians on these matters. A consensus suggests that experiments should be constructed so that there is less than a one in twenty chance (probability of .05) that there is no difference in the medical effects of the two treatments; that is, a sufficient number of subjects must be used so that there is a less than one in twenty chance that different results are due to coincidence or chance assignment rather than real differences in the treatments. The figure of .05 is admittedly somewhat arbitrary.

Many think that placebos are inert, mere "sugar pills." But this is not always the case. Placebos must be enough like the experimental treatment so that neither researchers nor subjects can tell the difference. For example, if the experimental treatment has drowsiness as a known side effect, then the placebo will have to produce drowsiness too to keep participants from figuring out who is in the control group and who is in the experimental group. As a result, some placebos must be quite invasive. Providing a detailed example will help.

In this case, researchers were working on the possible beneficial effects of cryogenic therapy—treating disease by lowering the temperature of all or part of the body.[13] Peptic ulcers—lesions in the stomach wall caused by excess gastric secretion of acid—were among the diseases being studied. A technique called "gastric freezing" was developed. This involved the insertion of a tube in the stomach. A balloon at the end of the tube contained a cold liquid that circulated and thereby lowered the temperature of the stomach. After being successful on dogs, the procedure was tried on patients who had been admitted to the hospital for surgical treatment of peptic ulcers. Thirty-one patients received the gastric freeze, a treatment lasting about one hour. All patients reported a marked or complete relief of stomach pain. This treatment was promising because it was much less dangerous or invasive than surgery.[14] In the years immediately following this report, gastric freezing was introduced in many hospitals. Patients began to report complications and physicians began to question the efficacy of the treatment. Still, a number of patients continued to report improvements.

Given the ambiguity of the evidence, a controlled trial of gastric freezing was needed to determine whether the improvements were due merely to the placebo effect. One group of patients would have to receive the real treatment and the other a placebo that resembles gastric freezing so that neither patients nor physicians would know who was in which group. To achieve this, researchers designed a tube and balloon that was like the gastric freeze equipment except that the cold liquid did not circulate in the balloon. In this sham procedure, patients felt cold in their mouths and throats, but the stomach was not cooled. Clearly the placebo in this case was invasive, not a mere sugar pill. The study, by the way, demonstrated that gastric freezing was no better than the sham in treating peptic ulcers.

Many ethical issues can be raised about RCTs. One key issue concerns whether subjects can be fully informed.[15] For the sake of simplicity, assume that the issue of informed consent can be adequately handled. Here, we shall discuss briefly two questions: When is it morally appropriate to initiate a RCT? Is it ever appropriate to stop a RCT that demonstrates promise and give all of the subjects the experimental treatment *before* a statistically significant result has been achieved?

Regarding the question about the appropriateness of initiating an RCT, let us make some modest observations.[16] First, if no treatment for the problem in question is available and if the subjects are not likely to be made worse off by participating in the trial than by not doing so, then initiating the trial is permissible. Second, if a treatment is available that is somewhat efficacious and that treatment is given to those in the control group, then no participant is knowingly made worse off and so the trial is permissible. The idea is that in each of these two cases, some promise of benefits exists, and no subject is knowingly made worse off than he would have been in not participating.

Two other cases are more troubling, however. First, if a standard treatment is available that is somewhat successful but some subjects are receiving a mere placebo, then this is morally problematic because some are knowingly made worse off than they would have been had they not participated, assuming that those who do not participate will receive the standard treatment. Second, if no standard treatment is available and the placebo makes subjects worse off than they would have been by not participating, then the trial is morally problematic. This second kind of case is illustrated in the gastric freeze study. Those receiving the sham treatment were made worse off because of the invasiveness of the treatment and its absence of medicinal benefits. Like some of the nontherapeutic experiments discussed earlier, however, this is somewhat complicated. For a utilitarian might argue that the discomfort experienced by the subjects is more than outweighed by the benefits that future patients will receive. In the gastric freeze case, many future patients (who knows how many?) will be spared the invasiveness of a procedure that produces no medical benefits. So again we have a case where the good of future patients can be promoted only by sacrificing the interests of current subjects.

The second issue concerns the appropriateness of stopping an RCT before statistical significance has been achieved and giving the experimental treatment to all subjects if that treatment looks promising. This issue arises repeatedly when, based on phase II trials, drugs appear promising in the fight against AIDS. Many AIDS activists demand that scientific rigors be relaxed and that promising drugs be made available to anyone who wants them.

An example of this dispute was explained on the television program *60 Minutes* (May 9, 1993). An experimental drug, called CNTF, has shown some promise in stopping the progression of amyotrophic lateral sclerosis (ALS), more commonly known as Lou Gehrig's disease. ALS is terminal and incurable. It results in the degeneration of motor neurons of the spinal cord, ultimately leading to death. The disease is progressively disabling. CNTF is undergoing a trial, testing its effectiveness at slowing the progress of ALS. The trial gives rise to two issues. First, merely being allowed to participate in the trial is a benefit. Access to the trial is, in effect, a scarce resource. (This issue will be discussed in Chapter 7.) Second, and more pertinent here, those participating in the study have a one-in-three chance of receiving a placebo. Many afflicted with ALS demand that all who want CNTF be granted access. Forget the study! What can be said in response to such demands, demands made by persons facing a death sentence?

RCTs should be carried out until statistical significance is achieved for at least two reasons—in spite of the pleas of the afflicted. First, health care professionals have an obligation not to present as routine treatment that which has not been adequately tested. To deviate from this obligation is to put the reputation of the health care profession at risk. This conservative approach to doling out treatment should actually enhance our trust in health care providers. But suppose that patients afflicted with a terrible illness, such as AIDS or ALS, agree to take the risk. They are informed, they understand that the treatment has not been fully tested, but they are understandably willing to incur the risk.

A second reason that RCTs should be carried out to their conclusions concerns the well-being of future patients. Mistakes can be made when we "jump the gun" and act too quickly. The experience with gastric freezing demonstrates that patients can be subjected to discomfort for no good medical reason. Moreover, progress in establishing a cure is slowed if trials are not completed. Even if what is being tested is not "the cure," completion of the trial may give researchers important clues that will hasten progress and help future patients.

You might think that researchers could make promising drugs available to many persons while going on to complete the RCT. But this would give rise to an obvious problem. As Lawrence Schneiderman and Nancy Jecker put it, "Sanctioning dubious drugs before their therapeutic efficacy is established by careful clinical trials only *delays* the discovery of useful drugs, because it makes recruitment of patients into prospective clinical trials more difficult."[17] Perhaps exceptions should be made. Absolute pronouncements in any of these areas are apt to be simplistic. But there are good reasons for completing RCTs before a treatment is made available to all.

An interesting twist occurs if the patient's physician is not a direct part of the research team. Physician Abraham Verghese, in his moving story about treating AIDS patients in eastern Tennessee, tells of sending a patient to Duke University for AZT trials on early HIV infection.[18] Duke entered the patient into a placebo-controlled RCT. One month after enrollment, Verghese recognized that his patient was receiving a placebo because of the absence of characteristic changes of red blood cells that AZT induces. Because his patient had to make a long and exhausting five-hour drive for each "treatment," Verghese was tempted to tell him that he was on a placebo and not to bother returning. He did not tell him, though eventually the patient figured it out for himself and dropped out of the study.

This discussion does not exhaust what there is to say about initiating RCT, or certainly what there is to say about RCTs in general. But we have a sketch of some of the main issues.

RESEARCH INVOLVING CHILDREN

We are suspicious about using children as experimental subjects, with good reason. Unlike adults, many children are not able to defend themselves or to understand what is in their long-run best interests. Moreover, because many of the capacities that children have are undeveloped, the risks involved in using them as subjects seem greater. Two sorts of risks come to mind. First, the chance that they will suffer irreparable physical harm seems greater than in the case of adults. Second, worries about the possibility of psychological or emotional harm that might be done to the child-subject are also common.

Nevertheless, to advocate an absolute prohibition on the use of children as experimental subjects is to go too far. There are biological differences between children and adults, differences in anatomy, metabolism, and the like. Consequently, certain drugs and treatments will have different effects on children than on adults. And to determine proper dosages for children, children must be used as subjects. In addition, children are subject to some diseases not prevalent among adults. Thus, if advances in treating children are to be made, they must be used in experiments. This point explains the rationale underlying the pronouncement in the AMA Ethical Guidelines for Clinical Investigation concerning the use of children as subjects. The guidelines do not absolutely prohibit the use of children, but before they may be used it must be certain that adults could not be used as suitable subjects. Given our hesitancy about using children and yet given the necessity of sometimes doing so, the position taken in the AMA guidelines seems quite plausible.

The Willowbrook State Hospital Case

Willowbrook State Hospital is an institution on Staten Island, New York, that houses and treats mentally retarded children.[19] The population at Willowbrook in 1949 was approximately 200. In 1972, there were 5,200 residents, of whom 3,800 were severely retarded. Hepatitis was detected among some of the residents at Willowbrook in 1949. Five years later, Dr. Saul Krugman was appointed as a consultant in pediatrics and infectious diseases. Infectious diseases were prevalent at Willowbrook; among them were hepatitis, measles, shigellosis, parasitic infections, and respiratory infections. Krugman and his associates, Drs. Joan Giles and Jack Hammond, initiated studies on hepatitis. Because many of the severely retarded children were not toilet-trained and because infectious hepatitis is transmitted by way of the intestinal-oral route, nearly all susceptible children admitted to Willowbrook became infected within the first year.

Between 1956 and 1970, approximately 10,000 children were admitted to the Willowbrook Hospital. Of those, 750 to 800 were admitted to the research unit of Krugman, Giles, and Hammond. The researchers injected these children-subjects with infected serum to produce in them a strain of hepatitis already prevalent at Willowbrook. The researchers' goals were to obtain a better understanding of hepatitis and to develop some methods of immunizing against it. Only children whose parents gave written consent were used as subjects.

In the early 1970s, this research was widely and critically discussed. Krugman, Giles, and Hammond, however, argued that no wrong was done and made a number of specific points in defense of the hepatitis research. First, they pointed out that the children used as subjects were made no worse off than they would have been in the natural conditions existing at Willowbrook, because virtually all of the children contracted hepatitis. Second, they argued that in some respects the children in their research unit benefited. Because they were being admitted to a special, well-equipped, and well-staffed unit, they would while in the unit be isolated from other infectious diseases so prevalent at Willowbrook. Moreover, it would be better to contract hepatitis under these highly controlled conditions. Third, as a result of being infected with a milder form of hepatitis, these children would be protected against more damaging forms of that disease by developing immunity. And fourth, they argued that only children whose parents gave informed consent were used as subjects. It should also be noted that the value of this research was recognized as significant in furthering our understanding of hepatitis.

Classical utilitarian elements are present in the defense offered by Krugman, Giles, and Hammond. They claimed that the children were made no worse off by their participation, that in fact they benefited, that society was likely to benefit from the growth of knowledge and improvements in the treatment of hepatitis, and that the fully informed consent of the parents was obtained. Like the researchers involved in the case at the Jewish Chronic Disease Hospital, these scientists argued, in effect, that the experiments were therapeutic in nature and that informed consent had been obtained. Utilitarian considerations were introduced as a backup. Because of the difficulty of justifying nontherapeutic experimentation without consent, it is not surprising that these doctors denied that they were engaged in such research.

Many in the medical community were outraged upon learning about the nature of this research. Objections were raised; a few of the principal ones will be explained here.

First, critics pointed out that this experiment was not therapeutic. Any benefits that the children-subjects received—such as isolation from other infectious diseases—were incidental. In no way was the chief aim of this research to benefit the children who were the subjects; rather, the main aim was to benefit future patients. There is also some debate about how great the benefits to society were likely to be. Paul Ramsey, for example, has argued that the research was merely designed to duplicate and confirm the efficacy of gamma globulin in immunization against hepatitis. What these researchers really wanted to do, Ramsey argued, was simply to develop further and improve on that inoculum.[20] Whether Ramsey is correct is not clear. But even if he is, these goals may be well worth pursuing. So from a utilitarian perspective, many positive things may be said about this case. The fact remains, however, that this research is better labeled "nontherapeutic."

Second, some have charged that though the parents of the children did agree to their participation, this consent was not freely given. An element of coercion or pressure was detected.[21] The charge here is that in later years when parents applied for admission to Willowbrook for their children, they would receive a form letter stating that no space was available. Shortly thereafter these parents would receive a letter indicating that there were some spaces available in the hepatitis research unit. So if the parents were willing to consent to allowing their children to be used as subjects in this research, the children would be admitted to Willowbrook; otherwise, not. This situation put parents in an untenable position. To receive institutionalization for their severely retarded children, they had to agree to allow them to serve as experimental subjects. Such consent is tainted.

Third, some argued that mentally retarded children should never be used as subjects because the possibility of abuse is much greater than it is when competent adults are used as subjects. According to these critics, even if the parents did consent, these children should not be used. Could not competent adults have served equally well as subjects, they asked? Some say, however, that in this case children were more suitable than adults to be subjects because hepatitis is much milder in persons in the three- to ten-year age group than in older individuals. And most of the children at Willowbrook were going to contract hepatitis anyway.

Questions were also raised about withholding from the general population at Willowbrook an inoculation known to have some degree of efficacy.[22] At some point during this study, the researchers knew that those from whom the gamma globulin was withheld were in more danger than the experimental subjects. This must be true if, as Krugman et al. claimed, the subjects benefited by getting a milder form of hepatitis followed by protection against more severe forms. This point suggests that those who were part of the general population at Willowbrook were being treated as a means only. They were being placed in a situation that was more risky than need be. This concern raises questions discussed earlier in the section on RCTs. To confirm the efficacy of a given treatment, a control group is needed from whom the treatment is withheld. But do we reach a point when continuing to withhold such treatment is unfair?

A situation like this occurred in 1960 with the development of the polio vaccine.[23] Drs. Weller, Enders, and Robbins had what they thought was an effective vaccine. But to satisfy the demands of scientific rigor, they needed a control group from whom this vaccine was withheld. So approximately 30,000 children were injected with a substance known to be useless in the prevention of polio. The researchers believed that some of these children would contract polio and die as a result, but this was the only way to confirm the effectiveness of the vaccine. The justification for imposing such serious risks on nonconsenting human subjects is utilitarian: enormous good for millions of people was the promise of this research. So we face again the conflict between the good of the whole and the rights of particular individuals.

Let us discuss one other objection that was raised against the research at Willowbrook. Recall that Krugman et al. claimed that their subjects actually benefited from participating in this study. And in some sense this claim seems correct. The children did receive additional attention and protection from other diseases prevalent at Willowbrook. But the only reason that they benefited was because conditions at Willowbrook were horrendous; almost anything would be an improvement. This fact casts a pall over the claim that the subjects benefited. It seems that the researchers took advantage of the children, just as researchers in the past took advantage of prisoners. What they should do instead, some claim, is to work to improve these conditions. One critic put it this way: "The duty of a pediatrician in a situation such as exists at Willowbrook State School is to attempt to improve that situation, not to turn it to his advantage for experimental purposes, however lofty the aims."[24] The critic's claim is that these physicians should be addressing fundamental problems, such as why infectious diseases were so prevalent at Willowbrook.

This last objection raises the more general issue of what obligations agents have in situations that are less than ideal. Two fundamentally different schools of thought prevail on this topic.[25] The view of the critic is a morally rigorous position, one that an idealist might adopt. Advocates of this view argue that any health care practitioner who encounters bad conditions, such as those at Willowbrook, should work to improve those conditions, not take advantage of persons trapped in them. Maybe not everyone owes a general duty of beneficence to strangers. But health care professionals who have the skills needed to improve the conditions and who have a special relationship with those who are suffering, as was the case with the researchers at Willowbrook, do have such a duty.

The other view, adopted by those who are inclined to defend the Willowbrook researchers against this objection, is more pragmatic; it is based on utilitarianism. According to this position, it is unrealistic to demand of researchers that they change all of the bad social conditions they might encounter. It is appropriate, instead, that they make the best of a bad situation. Unfortunately, some are so bad off that they might actually benefit by becoming subjects in experiments like those conducted at Willowbrook. But when that is the case, tradeoffs are appropriate. People will be given certain benefits in exchange for granting to researchers the privilege of using them as subjects. No one can change the world overnight. Improvements will be gradual, and many will ensue from knowledge gained during scientific research; this is the best individuals can do.

SUMMARY

Nontherapeutic experiments do not benefit subjects directly; their aim is to produce knowledge that will help future patients. A goal of this chapter was to discuss the moral limitations on such research. Three types of nontherapeutic experiments are morally troubling: those in which subjects have given informed consent but are at risk, those in which subjects are not at risk but have not given informed consent, and those in which subjects are at risk and have not given informed consent. The grounds for supporting and opposing each of these types of experiments were discussed, with examples.

Random clinical trials are common in scientific research today. Because they involve control groups that may receive placebos and because assignment to treatment is random, moral issues arise concerning the initiation of such studies. Another problem concerns the premature termination of RCTs. This issue is especially pressing when the early data indicate that the experimental treatment is successful and would benefit all participants. It is also critical when the preliminary data suggest that the treatment is not successful, though that result was not discussed here.

Using children as experimental subjects is troubling but sometimes necessary. As the Willowbrook State Hospital case illustrates, children who are research subjects are sometimes put at risk. Such research raises many moral issues, including whether the possible benefits for society outweigh the risks imposed on the subjects, whether the risks are greater than the subjects would otherwise encounter, whether researchers are inappropriately taking advantage of the subjects, and whether the subjects' guardians gave genuine consent.

From the cases at the Jewish Chronic Disease Hospital and the Willowbrook State School, three important results have been lasting. First, for research to be therapeutic, its principal aim must be to benefit the subjects. Mere beneficial side effects do not render a study therapeutic. Second, for consent to be fully informed, researchers must give to subjects or their legal guardians all information about the study. Researchers may not exclude information that they think is irrelevant but would prompt subjects to refuse to participate. Finally, for consent to be freely given, no coercion or pressure may be exerted on the subjects or legal guardians. Making participation in an experiment a condition of hospital admission or the receipt of treatment is unacceptable.

Suggestions for Further Reading

Coppenger, Mark. *Bioethics: A Casebook* (Upper Saddle River, NJ: Prentice Hall, 1985), Chapter 4.

Erwin, Edward, Sidney Gendin, and Lowell Kleiman (eds.). *Ethical Issues in Scientific Research* (New York: Garland, 1994).

Jones, James H. *Bad Blood: The Tuskegee Syphilis Experiment*, rev. ed. (New York: Free Press, 1993).

Levine, Robert J. *Ethics and Regulation of Clinical Research* (New Haven, CT: Yale University Press, 1986).

Miller, Bruce. "Experimentation on Human Subjects: The Ethics of Random Clinical Trials." In Donald VanDeVeer and Tom Regan (eds.), *Health Care Ethics* (Philadelphia: Temple University Press, 1987), pp. 127–159.

Munson, Ronald (ed.). *Intervention and Reflection: Basic Issues in Medical Ethics*, 4th ed. (Belmont, CA: Wadsworth, 1992), Chapter 6.

Pence, Gregory E. *Classic Cases in Medical Ethics* (New York: McGraw-Hill, 1990), Chapters 8–12.

Ramsey, Paul. *The Patient as Person* (New Haven, CT: Yale University Press, 1970), Chapter 1.

Rothman, Kenneth J., and Karin B. Michels. "The Continuing Unethical Use of Placebo Controls." *New England Journal of Medicine*, Vol. 331 (1994), pp. 394–398.

Silverman, William A. *Human Experimentation* (New York: Oxford University Press, 1985), Chapter 12.

Veatch, Robert M. *Case Studies in Medical Ethics* (Cambridge, MA: Harvard University Press, 1977), Chapter 11.

Notes

1. See Franz J. Ingelfinger, "Informed (But Uneducated) Consent," in Ronald Munson (ed.), *Intervention and Reflection: Basic Issues in Medical Ethics*, 4th ed. (Belmont, CA: Wadsworth, 1992), pp. 355–357.

2. Robert M. Veatch, *Case Studies in Medical Ethics* (Cambridge, MA: Harvard University Press, 1977), pp. 271–273.

3. Terrence F. Ackerman and Carson Strong, *A Casebook of Medical Ethics* (New York: Oxford University Press, 1989), pp. 153–155.

4. For a discussion of this case, see Elinor Langer, "Human Experimentation: New York Verdict Affirms Patient's Rights," *Science* 151: 11, pp. 663–666, and Mark Coppenger, *Bioethics: A Casebook* (Upper Saddle River, NJ: Prentice Hall, 1985), pp. 105–106.

5. This point is made sardonically by Preston J. Burnham in "Medical Experimentation on Humans," *Science* 152: 22, pp. 448–450.

6. Ackerman and Strong, *A Casebook of Medical Ethics*, pp. 135–137.

7. For a detailed account of this, see James H. Jones, *Bad Blood*, rev. ed. (New York: Free Press, 1993). See also Gregory E. Pence, *Classic Cases in Medical Ethics* (New York: McGraw-Hill, 1990), Chapter 9.

8. R. A. Vonderlehr, T. Clark, and J. R. Heller, "Untreated Syphilis in the Male Negro," *Journal of the American Medical Association* 107 (September 12, 1936), pp. 856–860.

9. See Ruth Faden (ed.), *The Human Radiation Experiments* (New York: Oxford University Press, 1996).

10. Veatch, *Case Studies in Medical Ethics*, pp. 299–302.

11. Veatch, *Case Studies in Medical Ethics*, p. 302.

12. For an excellent discussion of random clinical trials, from which this discussion borrows heavily, see Bruce Miller, "Experimentation on Human Subjects: The Ethics of Random Clinical Trials," in Donald VanDeVeer and Tom Regan (eds.), *Health Care Ethics* (Philadelphia: Temple University Press, 1987), pp. 127–159.

13. This case is explained in Miller, "Experimentation on Human Subjects," pp. 132–134.

14. Reported in O. H. Wangensteen, E. T. Peter, D. M. Nicoloff, A. I. Walder, H. Sosin, and E. F. Berstein, "Achieving 'Physiological Gastrectomy' by Gastric Freezing," *Journal of the American Medical Association* 180 (1962), pp. 439–444.

15. See Miller, "Experimentation on Human Subjects," pp. 137–138.

16. For a much more thorough discussion of these and related issues, see Miller, "Experimentation on Human Subjects," pp. 143–157. See also Kenneth J. Rothman and Karin B. Michels, "The Continuing Unethical Use of Placebo Controls," *New England Journal of Medicine*, Vol. 331 (1994), pp. 394–398.

17. Lawrence Schneiderman and Nancy Jecker, *Wrong Medicine: Doctors, Patients, and Futile Treatment* (Baltimore: Johns Hopkins University Press, 1995), p. 169.

18. Abraham Verghese, *My Own Country* (New York: Simon & Schuster, 1994), p. 245.

19. This case is widely discussed in the literature on experimentation. See Veatch, *Case Studies in Medical Ethics*, pp. 274–275; Tom L. Beauchamp and James F. Childress, *Principles of Biomedical Ethics*, 4th ed. (New York: Oxford University Press, 1994), pp. 519–522; Munson (ed.), *Intervention and Reflection: Basic Issues in Medical Ethics*, pp. 312–314, 367–370; and Paul Ramsey, *The Patient as Person* (New Haven, CT: Yale University Press, 1970), pp. 47–58.

20. Ramsey, *The Patient as Person*, p. 47.

21. Ramsey, *The Patient as Person*, pp. 53–54.

22. Ramsey, *The Patient as Person*, p. 49.

23. Munson, *Intervention and Reflection*, pp. 325–326.

24. Stephen Goldby, "Letters," in Munson (ed.), *Intervention and Reflection*, p. 368.

25. These positions are discussed, though in a somewhat different way from my approach, in Veatch, *Case Studies in Medical Ethics*, p. 277.

CHAPTER 7

Allocating and Obtaining Scarce Medical Resources

MANY MEDICAL RESOURCES are potentially scarce, including medical machinery such as ventilators and dialysis units, drugs, blood, organs for transplantation, space in an intensive care unit, or the time of the health care practitioner, such as in situations of triage. As recent developments have shown, even the privilege of being a subject in a medical experiment may be a scarce resource. In 1993, for example, a hospital in Greensboro, North Carolina, began participating in an experiment (along with fifteen other medical centers throughout the United States) testing a vaccine for patients who have a virus that causes AIDS (HIV). Suitable subjects are persons who have the virus but do not yet show symptoms of AIDS. Obviously anyone who is already HIV positive would like to be in this test; yet, only thirteen people with HIV can be admitted.[1]

When the demand for medical resources is greater than the supply, difficult moral problems emerge. Two in particular stand out. First, as long as the supply of a given resource is inadequate, to whom do we allocate it? Second, what should we do to increase the supply?

Both of these issues concern matters of social policy. These are not problems that a few individuals, acting on their own, can solve. Rather, they must be addressed by society collectively. Society must have policies about allocating scarce medical resources and obtaining additional resources. In this chapter, the major proposals that have been advanced will be examined.

Medical resources can be divided into two types, *human* resources and *nonhuman* resources. Human resources are obtained directly from the

214

bodies of human beings. Examples include blood, bone marrow, and organs for transplantation, such as kidneys, livers, lungs, and hearts. Nonhuman medical resources either are made by human beings or are found in nature. Examples include drugs, artificial organs, respirators, dialysis units, and the like. When discussing the issue of *allocating* scarce medical resources, this distinction may not be important. It seems that the same principles should apply whether the scarce resource to be distributed is human or nonhuman. When addressing how best to *obtain* scarce medical resources, however, the distinction does seem significant. Making nonhuman medical resources more plentiful seems to be a matter of spending more time and money and developing more ingenuity. Since this process likely involves the use of public money, it raises important issues of distributive justice. Indeed, much debate involves whether more resources should be put into programs for AIDS, breast cancer, prenatal care, preventive medicine, and the like. In effect, these groups are competing for bigger pieces of the same pie. Here, however, the focus will be on the assessment of policies used to obtain human medical resources.

We begin with the issue of allocation.

ALLOCATING SCARCE MEDICAL RESOURCES

When the demand or need for a medical resource exceeds the available supply, several moral questions are raised. Who among the candidates shall receive the scarce resource? Who will make these decisions? And what criterion or criteria should be used in deciding who receives the scarce resource? The question about who decides is important. Should the decision be made by physicians, all of the health care professionals involved, or a committee made up in part by laypersons? The decisions in these cases are moral, not purely medical. Recognition that some decisions made in medical contexts are moral explains, in part, why many hospitals have formed ethics committees, composed of some laypersons, to address such issues. Still, one suspects that the question about what criteria should be employed is the most important one, and that concern will be the focus of this section.

One might be tempted to think that the problem of allocating scarce medical resources will disappear when technology becomes sufficiently advanced. This view is a mistake, however. Given the nature of advancement in medicine, there will always be scarce resources. When new discoveries are made, typically the resource in question is expensive and difficult to produce. Improvements may be made with respect to that resource, so that it is no longer in scarce supply; but then another new resource will come along. Depending on the society and its stage of development, the scarce resources may be penicillin, dialysis units, blood, organs for transplantation, the time that health care professionals have for their patients, and who knows what in the future. Though any particular good may go from scarce to plentiful supply, the general moral problem is likely always to exist.

Two competing theories for allocating scarce medical resources will be described here. One of these theories appeals to considerations of utility and the social worth of the candidates. According to this view, society should regard the allocation of scarce medical resources as an investment on which it seeks to maximize its return. Allocating scarce resources to those who are most likely to make valuable contributions to society is likely the best way to maximize the return on the investment. Thus, advocates of this theory might maintain that physicians should be saved before common laborers, that nurses should receive treatment before maids, and that engineers should be selected ahead of barbers. The competing theory for allocating scarce medical resources is called the lottery method. According to this view, each person should have an equal opportunity to receive the scarce medical resource. This end is best achieved by letting luck determine which candidates will be selected to receive the resource in question. Each of these theories will be examined in detail later.

An Example

To begin, let us consider an actual case in which a committee was formed for the express purpose of allocating a scarce medical resource. This case took place at the Swedish Hospital in Seattle, Washington, in 1962.[2] Access to dialysis for victims of kidney failure was the scarce resource in this case. The number of persons who sought access to these units was far greater than the available supply at the Swedish Hospital. A committee of laypersons was formed to choose among the applicants. Members of the committee remained anonymous to protect them from public pressures. An effort was made to have different elements of the community represented on the committee. In 1963, for example, the committee was composed of two physicians, a banker, a lawyer, a homemaker, a labor leader, and a member of the clergy. The idea underlying this sort of representation was presumably to prevent skewed or prejudicial judgments that might result if only a few segments of the community were involved. Given the sort of decisions that were to be made, many referred to this as a life-or-death committee.

From what we know, it appears that the committee adopted a version of the theory that distributes scarce resources on the basis of utility and the social worth of the candidates. Before appealing to any notion of social worth, however, the committee took two other factors into account. On the advice of physicians, persons over forty-five years old and very young children were excluded from consideration. These individuals, it was thought, would not respond well to dialysis. Children, for example, may not mature physically and may have a difficult time sticking to the regimen. The committee also gave priority to residents of the state of Washington. Because the hospital received much of its funding from state taxes, it was thought that Washingtonians were especially entitled to the benefits of the hospital.

Of the remaining candidates, the persons selected seemed to be those thought to have the greatest social worth. Exactly how social worth was determined remains unclear. We do know, however, what sort of information the committee requested. They wanted to know the following about each of the prospective patients: age, gender, marital status, number of dependents, income, emotional stability (especially the patient's capacity to tolerate treatment), occupation, educational background, past performances, and future potential.[3] The committee was not told the names of the candidates so as to avoid the charge of personal favoritism or bias. The information that the committee requested was conveyed by the patient's physician. Bits and pieces of the committee's deliberations have been reported. It is claimed that the committee looked favorably on those who played an active role in a church. Some members apparently thought that this was an indication of moral strength. And apparently the committee gave preference to persons with many dependents and those who were poor.

The work of the Swedish Hospital committee has been widely criticized.[4] The most common objections that were raised will be explained here. First, the case for each patient was made by his physician. Of course, some people write better and argue more persuasively than others. As a result, how convincingly a patient's physician could write greatly affected that patient's chances of being selected by the committee. Moreover, some people are inclined to exaggerate when they play the role of an advocate, while others will be scrupulously honest. And the critics think that clearly these factors should not play a role in determining whether a patient receives a scarce medical resource. Patients do not select doctors because they write well, argue persuasively, or are inclined to exaggerate.

Second, some critics maintain that any such committee will inevitably promote middle-class values. What underlies this criticism is the belief that our knowledge of social worth is limited and that most of the criteria that have been proposed are unpersuasive. One author sardonically noted that a patient coming before the Swedish Hospital committee would do well to sire a great number of children and to give away all of his money. Others quipped that a nonconformist such as Henry David Thoreau would not fare well if he lived in Seattle and had bad kidneys.[5] History is fraught with examples where a person's contemporaries castigated her, and only later generations appreciated the person's true worth.

Finally, some argued that the very fact that human beings were selecting some to be saved and rejecting others is an instance of people "playing God." Each person possesses an equal right to life and an equal right to the medical necessities to maintain life. When human beings deliberately select some and reject others on the basis of perceived social worth, they violate this equality. So, the critics maintain, introducing the notion of social worth in the context of allocating scarce medical resources is unwarranted. Before dismissing completely the social worth theory, however, it is advisable to examine a more detailed version of it.

Rescher's Theory of Social Worth

In spite of the objections to the work of the Swedish Hospital committee, some have thought that consequentialist considerations in general and social worth in particular must play a role in deciding who will receive scarce medical resources. Consequentialist factors are definitely invoked in some medical contexts. For example, in allocating money to fund research projects, a relevant consideration is how many will be helped if the research is successful. So perhaps similar considerations should be invoked in determining who should receive scarce medical resources.

Nicholas Rescher defends an approach to this issue that is based on consequentialism and appeals to the notion of social worth.[6] Rescher divides the process of selecting recipients of scarce medical resources into two stages. The first stage is designed to narrow the field of applicants to a workable number. To accomplish this, what Rescher calls *criteria of inclusion* must be formulated. Persons who do not satisfy at least some of the criteria will be excluded; they will not qualify as suitable recipients. Persons who do satisfy at least some of the criteria will be considered at the second stage; they are serious candidates.

A nonmedical example can be used to explain how criteria of inclusion work. Consider the admissions policy of a university. If, as is true of the best universities, a school receives far more applications than it has positions available, it is not feasible to examine carefully the credentials of each applicant. So such a university may have certain requirements that function as criteria of inclusion. It may, for example, routinely deny admission to anyone who scores below a certain level on the entrance examination. Or it may reject any student whose high school grade point average falls below a certain fixed mark. Employing such procedures then allows universities to examine the records of students who satisfy these initial criteria very carefully, on a case-by-case basis.

When the field of applicants has been narrowed to a workable number, additional criteria are needed to decide who among the remaining candidates will receive the scarce resource. Rescher calls standards employed at this second stage *criteria of comparison*. To continue the previous analogy, a university's admissions committee might at this point examine the applicants' letters of recommendation, their extracurricular activities, and the like.

To narrow the field of applicants for a scarce medical resource, Rescher suggests three criteria of inclusion. Each criterion has a consequentialist rationale. The first of these is what Rescher calls the *constituency factor*. Often medical resources are available only in the institutional setting of a hospital. Sometimes hospitals or medical institutes have what might be called normal clientele boundaries; that is, some hospitals are set up to serve only certain patients, or at least to give priority to those individuals. Examples include veterans' hospitals, hospitals supported by funds from the state, and perhaps hospitals supported by churches. When allocating scarce medical resources, Rescher contends that an institution is justified in giving preference to those persons who are a part of its natural constituency. This is exactly what the Swedish Hospital did when it chose Washingtonians ahead of all others. One rationale for this practice is that those who are a part of the hospital's natural clientele have a special entitlement to that institution's resources. But there may be a deeper consequentialist defense of this criterion. Allowing institutions to give preference to their own clientele will encourage them to work harder because of the special satisfaction associated with taking care of "their own." If each institution works harder, the total supply of the resource in question is likely to be greater.

Suppose that the results of previous allocations show that a given scarce medical resource is effective only for a certain class of patients. Suppose, for example, that only women under the age of forty or persons with a certain blood type can be treated successfully with the resource in question. If this is the case, Rescher says that it is appropriate to give preference to those for whom the treatment is likely to be successful. This is the second criterion of inclusion, the *prospect of success factor*. This criterion too can be justified on consequentialist grounds. In allocating a scarce medical resource, society is making an investment; it should seek a favorable return. One obviously beneficial goal is saving as many lives as possible. This second criterion promotes that goal.

The third criterion of inclusion proposed by Rescher is the *progress of science factor*. Medical practitioners need to learn as much as they can about how various drugs and forms of treatment will affect future patients so that they can use them most efficiently. Certain medical resources may never have been given to certain types of patients or may have been given to so few that adequate data are unavailable. Therefore, learning how the resource in question will affect these patients is important. Such knowledge can guide future allocation decisions by refining the prospect-of-success factor. It may be useful, for example, to learn how very young children respond to a certain treatment or how successful a given drug is for elderly patients. Rescher says that this consideration may be taken into account in reducing the field of initial applicants; its potential consequentialist value for future patients is clear.

Let us now move to the second stage and examine the criteria of comparison. There are five in all; the first two are medical in nature, and the last three appeal to the notion of social worth. Again, these criteria have a consequentialist rationale. The first criterion of comparison is the *relative likelihood of success factor*, which is similar to the second criterion of inclusion. The difference is that this involves a case-by-case comparison. Two patients may fall in the same general category, yet the severity of one patient's problem may be greater than that of the other patient. If this is the case (and everything else is equal), then it makes sense to give the scarce medical resource to the patient who has the greater probability of being helped by it.

The *life expectancy factor* is the second criterion of comparison advocated by Rescher. This factor requires that patients' ages and other aspects of their medical condition (that is, aspects other than that which is to be treated by the scarce resource) be considered. Those who have a longer life expectancy are to be given preference. If one patient is twenty-five years old and another is sixty-five years old, and if the severity of the medical problem for each is the same, then the younger of the two should be given preference because that patient's life expectancy is greater. By the same reasoning, if each of two patients is similarly afflicted but one has an additional life-threatening problem, then the person without the additional complication should be given preference.

A consequentialist rationale supports these first two criteria of comparison. One of society's legitimate goals is to maximize the "life years" it receives from the investment of the scarce medical resource. These criteria promote that end by giving preference to patients who will benefit the most from receiving the resource.

The remaining criteria of comparison appeal to the notion of social worth. The third is what Rescher calls the *family role factor*. People are valuable to others as well as to themselves. In particular, the relationships between a person and her spouse, children, and parents are important. Often members of a person's immediate family are financially and/or emotionally dependent on that individual. Rescher argues that it is appropriate to take this into account when distributing exotic lifesaving treatment. If other things are equal, a mother with dependent children should be selected ahead of a middle-aged bachelor. Again, consequentialist considerations underlie this criterion. Society should benefit as many people as it can when it allocates its scarce medical resources. By giving preference to the mother over the bachelor, society benefits not only the mother but her children too. And indeed, by refusing to give preference to the mother, society may significantly harm the children.

The next criterion of comparison is the *potential future contributions factor*. Here we must try to determine what valuable services in the future each of the candidates is likely to render. In making such judgment, the candidates' ages, talents, level of education, and past record of performance must be taken into account. The consequentialist argument in support of this criterion is now familiar. Society is investing one of its valuable resources and is entitled to look for the best return on its investment. The optimal result is to allocate the resource in a way that will benefit the most people. Thus, this fourth criterion may require that a brilliant surgeon be chosen over a common laborer, and an experienced nurse ahead of a childless homemaker. Clearly such judgments are fallible. But, Rescher argues, that the judgments are difficult to make is not a reason for refusing to make them at all.

Finally, Rescher's fifth criterion of comparison is the *past services rendered factor,* which Rescher says is a necessary correlate of the factor of prospective service. Societies, like individuals, can incur debts of gratitude. If someone has worked long and hard for the good of society, that individual should be rewarded. Thus, society should give preference to those who have rendered significant services in the past when allocating scarce medical resources. In deciding whether to give a scarce resource to a lifelong criminal or a retired nurse, then, the latter should be chosen because of past services rendered. Even this factor is based on a forward-looking, consequentialist consideration: if society regularly rewards those who make valuable contributions, this practice will encourage others to make contributions.

This system, as presented so far, is not complete. Clearly, the five criteria of comparison can conflict. A method for handling potential conflicts is needed, and many options are possible. A hierarchial arrangement of the five criteria might be suggested. Thus, someone might propose that the relative likelihood of success factor is the most important and should take precedence over the other four, that the life expectancy factor is the second most important, and so forth. Rescher himself says that as long as all five of the factors are taken into account, many equally appropriate ways to resolve conflicts are possible. The method that he prefers is to give equal weight to the medical factors (that is, the likelihood of success and life expectancy) and the extramedical factors (that is, the three social considerations). Of course, if equal weight is given to each of these sets, then the possibility of a tie still exists. The candidate with the greatest likelihood of success may be a convicted criminal, and the patient who has rendered or probably will render the greatest services to society may have a much lower probability of recovery. When this point is reached, Rescher suggests that a method of random selection be employed. To use such a method at this stage has several advantages, according to Rescher. It will be perceived to be more fair, rejected patients will feel less bitter, and those who have to deal with these cases will be relieved of at least some difficult decisions.

This, then, is a brief sketch of a method of allocating scarce medical resources based on consequentialist considerations and in which the notion of social worth plays a key role. Whether this system avoids the criticisms that were directed at the Swedish Hospital committee is worth pondering. Some will say that the point regarding the promotion of middle-class values is still worrisome. When estimating likely future contributions, nonconformists are not apt to be treated well. Yet it is just such people who are often judged to be great when the verdict of history has been rendered. Some have also suggested that this system violates the fundamental belief in the equality of all people. The system wrongly suggests that a surgeon is a better person than a laborer. Whether plausible responses to these objections are possible is a matter for readers to consider. For now, let us turn to an alternative, one that purports to avoid these difficulties.

Childress's Lottery Method

Many reject the view that scarce medical resources should be allocated on the basis of consequentialist considerations or those of social worth. The very idea of deliberately selecting those persons who will be given a chance to live strikes some as wrong. The most popular alternative to the method of social worth is the lottery method. Defenders of this view advocate that who receives the scarce medical resource in question should be a matter of luck, not deliberate human choice. Such a method might be instituted in different ways. One way is to have an actual lottery; another is to adopt the policy "first come, first served." Under the latter system, whether a patient receives the scarce medical resource in question depends on when that patient needs it and how many others have already requested it, which are matters of luck.

The lottery method has been defended by several as the most appropriate way of allocating scarce medical resources. Here we will examine one defense of this method, advanced by James Childress.[7] Childress, like Rescher, recommends a two-step procedure. The first step, corresponding to Rescher's criteria of inclusion, is designed to reduce the field of applicants by appealing only to medical considerations: only those who can benefit medically from the receipt of the resource should advance to stage 2. The judgments made at this first stage are medical and should be made by those with medical expertise. That the judgments are medical rather than moral does not mean that they will necessarily be easy, however.

What determines whether a person is medically acceptable and is to be included among those to be considered at the second stage? Childress argues that candidates who have a reasonable prospect of responding positively to the treatment should be regarded as medically acceptable. What counts as a reasonable prospect of responding favorably to treatment is not easy to define. What Childress seems to have in mind is a rough judgment of common sense that the person has a good chance of benefiting medically if the treatment is administered. Childress also maintains that medical considerations should be employed *only* at this first stage. Once the second stage is reached, no finer distinctions on medical grounds should be used. Once it has been determined that each of two patients has a good chance of benefiting from the treatment in question, one should not be chosen over the other because of an even better chance of being helped. This approach contrasts sharply with Rescher's employment of medical criteria.

Candidates who will actually receive the scarce resource are selected at the second stage. Here Childress advocates that some version of the lottery method be used. Childress's argument has two parts: first, he raises several difficulties with the view that appeals to social worth; second, he cites positive considerations that support a method of random selection.

Any method that distributes scarce medical resources by appealing to social worth is defective, according to Childress. One problem is that our judgments about who is valuable to society change radically over the years. As noted earlier, persons like Socrates and Thoreau were denigrated by their contemporaries but now are regarded as great. Moreover, who is valuable to society depends on society's needs, and those needs are ever changing and difficult to predict. Just think of the various professions that you might pursue. For each of those, at one time it might be highly valued by society, at a later time not so highly valued. When people believe that our energy resources are virtually unlimited, geologists and petroleum engineers are not greatly valued; but when they believe that there is a crisis in our energy supply, such judgments are apt to be different. This first objection is pragmatic in nature; it says that we are not good judges of social worth.

Childress's second criticism is more of an "in principle" objection. It says that allocating scarce medical resources according to judgments about the candidates' social worth violates our belief in the equality of people. If we give priority to the surgeon over the laborer, we seem, in effect, to be saying that the surgeon is more valuable as a person, which is wrong.

There are also positive reasons for preferring the lottery method. First, unlike the method that appeals to social worth, the lottery method expresses our belief in the equality of people. What better way is there of expressing to candidates a belief in their equal worth than by providing for true equality of opportunity! Second, this method will do more than any of its competitors in promoting the relationship of trust between physicians and patients. Trust requires a belief that one will be dealt with fairly; and if in situations of scarcity resources are allocated by a method of random selection, then candidates can be confident that they have been treated impartially. Third, some think that the attitude of those who are not selected to receive the scarce medical resource will be better if the reason is the luck of the draw rather than that they are judged to lack social worth. It is one thing to lose because of bad luck; it is much more devastating to be told that you are unqualified. Finally, some speculate that the shortage of the resource in question is more apt to disappear if society uses the lottery method rather than that of social worth. In at least some cases, alleviating the shortage requires a greater commitment of society's resources. Those with wealth and in positions of power are the ones most likely to be in positions to effect such changes. Yet these are the very people who are likely to be chosen if scarce resources are allocated on the basis of social worth. Therefore, the argument goes, they will be more motivated to work for the elimination of the shortage if their chances of being a recipient are no greater than anyone else's.

Childress recommends that the best way to implement the method of random selection is for society to adopt the policy of "first come, first served." Under such a policy, persons who have passed the test of the first stage will be those whom physicians judge have a good chance of benefiting medically from the scarce resource in question. If that resource is available at that time, then the patients will be permitted to use it. If the resource is not available, then the candidates will be in line, as it were, awaiting their turn. Should the resource become available, the candidate is granted access to it.

Whether "first come, first served" is always the best way to implement the lottery method is debatable; perhaps it depends on the context and the resource to be distributed. But even when "first come, first served" is the best policy, a qualification is needed. We must add that in order for candidates to remain eligible to receive the resource, it must be the case that they can still benefit medically from its receipt. Without this qualification, a problem exists, at least when the policy concerns organ transplants. For those who rise to the top of the waiting list presumably have been waiting the longest, and through progressive deterioration over time they may be the least promising recipients of organ transplants.[8] Unless a suitable qualification is made, the very purpose of the first stage—admitting only those who are likely to benefit—will have been undermined.

Once the lottery method is understood, there is a temptation to look for exceptions, cases where a deliberate decision should be made instead of allowing the matter to be settled by chance. Childress himself is willing to allow for one exception. He suggests that it would be justifiable to give preferential treatment to someone who is practically indispensable to society, for example, the president during a grave national emergency. The difficulty, of course, is that allowing for one exception may open Pandora's box; once the first is allowed, many others will follow, and the merits of the lottery method will have been lost. In fact, the principle underlying the exception that Childress allows is used by critics of the lottery method.

The first criticism of this view is that in some situations employing a method of random selection is not advisable; these are situations in which deliberate choice is appropriate. Consider the following cases.[9] First, suppose that an emergency situation exists. Many people need medical assistance, but few are available to give it. In such a situation, one of the scarce resources is the time and energy of health care practitioners. Who should be treated first in these situations? Should some version of the lottery method be employed? Critics argue that it would be more rational to treat first those persons who can be restored quickly. These people will then be able to provide health care workers with additional assistance, even if they are laypersons. And if some of the people who need help are physicians and nurses, they should be given priority. This decision is not because they are better than others; rather, they can help in saving additional persons.

Another situation not medical in nature illustrates the same principle. Suppose that a number of persons are stranded at sea. There are too many for the lifeboat to support, so some must be thrown overboard or all will die. This situation, like the allocation of scarce medical resources, requires a life-or-death decision. Should the lottery method be used here? Again, critics have argued that in certain contexts it would be irrational to do so. Suppose that only one of the stranded persons is skilled in navigation. Without that person to serve as a guide, chances are good that no one will be saved. It would be foolish not to give preferential treatment to the navigator, not because the navigator is a better person but because her skills are needed if anyone is to be saved.

Consider a historical case.[10] In 1943, penicillin was in short supply for the U.S. Armed Forces in North Africa. Among the groups who could have benefited from its use were those who had venereal diseases and infected battle wounds. A decision had to be made concerning the allocation of penicillin. Some might think that the wounded should be given priority on moral grounds. But the officers in charge argued that those with venereal disease should be treated first because these persons could be restored to active duty more quickly, thus better enabling the group to achieve its purpose. Again, employing the lottery method would be unwise.

Another objection to the lottery method appeals to the merit of the candidates. First, some argue that in allocating scarce medical resources, we should not allow equal access to those who are responsible for their own medical problems. For example, we should not allow a lifelong smoker access to lungs for transplantation, and we should not allow a heavy drinker access to a liver transplant. If we allow equal access in cases like these, we fail to discourage unhealthy behavior. The second appeal to merit concerns the moral character of the candidates. If convicted mass murderers were among those who needed a scarce medical resource—say, an organ for transplantation—and would probably benefit from it, should society really allow them an equal opportunity to receive it? It is difficult to make comparative judgments of moral worth, and in most situations involving the allocation of a scarce medical resource, worth will not be a factor. But the extreme situations envisioned here are ones about which society may feel confident. Should merit not play a role, at least in these cases?

If these criticisms are persuasive, at least two alternatives are still possible. The lottery method can be rejected as unacceptable and some other method can be adopted instead, or exceptions can be made to the general policy that each medically suitable patient must be given an equal opportunity to receive the scarce medical resource in question. The difficulty with the latter move is that there must be a *principled* basis for allowing such exceptions. Moreover, this principled basis cannot appeal to social worth; for if that is the basis, advocates of the lottery method will have conceded too much to defenders of the social worth theory.

The two views discussed here—the social worth theory and the lottery method—are the most widely held policies for distributing scarce medical resources. Only one other position has received much notice: when not all can be saved, no one should be saved.[11] (Reportedly, J. M. Keynes called this the *principle of equal unfairness*.) But this view has few advocates and does not seem plausible. The moral problem of how to allocate scarce medical resources is especially troublesome because it is unavoidable, and criticisms of the two major positions have a ring of plausibility. We must deal with these issues, yet the usual ways of doing so seem inadequate.

We conclude this section with a particular example. In 1993, Robert Casey, governor of Pennsylvania, was diagnosed as having amyloidosis. Governor Casey's disease was life-threatening; the afflicted organ was the liver. He underwent tests to determine whether he was a suitable candidate for a liver transplant. His heart was determined to be too weak, and his only hope was to undergo a heart and liver transplant. He underwent this procedure in June 1993.

Two things about this case are worthy of discussion. First, Governor Casey was on the waiting list for a heart and liver transplant for *only one day.* The time potential recipients spend on a waiting list varies radically and depends on many factors, including, of course, the availability of a suitable donor. Nevertheless, some wonder whether Governor Casey "jumped the queue" and was given special consideration because of his position. Second, at the time of Governor Casey's surgery, fewer than ten heart and liver transplants had been performed. As a result, this procedure was highly experimental; its success rate was not well known. Because of this concern, some wondered whether these organs might not have been put to better use if distributed to other needy recipients. The critics' point is that from a consequentialist perspective it might have made more sense to give the liver to one person, the heart to another, and so forth, because the chances of saving each of these persons are likely greater than the chances of saving the governor. These and other questions about this case may be discussed in light of the two theories outlined here.

OBTAINING SCARCE MEDICAL RESOURCES

If lifesaving resources are scarce, society must do what it can to increase the supply. We therefore must ask what policy options society has with respect to obtaining the various resources and which will work best. Here we shall examine policies for acquiring cadaver organs for transplantation and policies for acquiring renewable medical resources, such as blood.

Obtaining Cadaver Organs

Since the advent of transplantation, cadaver organs have been valuable medical resources. Now hearts, lungs, livers, pancreases, kidneys, and other organs from the newly dead can be used to save lives. In the United States, we rely principally on donations to obtain cadaver organs. But this system is not working well. At the present time, more than 30,000 people in the United States are waiting for organs for transplantation. Approximately 2,500 people die each year waiting for organs.[12] Some, especially those needing a kidney transplant, have been on the waiting list for years. And the problem is even worse than these figures suggest; for many potential recipients are not even placed on waiting lists by their physicians.[13]

Of course, not everyone who dies is a medically suitable donor; indeed, the pool is small. For those who die from chronic and debilitating diseases and the elderly are not likely to be good donors, except possibly for parts of the eye. Lori Brigham, executive director of the Washington Regional Transplant Consortium, says that potentially medically suitable cadaver organ donors come from a pool of 15,000 to 20,000 newly deceased, most of whom have died from automobile accidents and head injuries. Yet the actual number of donors per year is approximately 4,000.[14] This shortage is even more profound among African-American citizens. Blacks, who make up approximately 12 percent of the U.S. population, account for 30 percent of the persons waiting for organ transplants. Dr. Clive Callender, director of the Howard University Hospital Transplant Center, explains this disparity: "Transplants in black patients are less successful than in white patients, partially because good organ matches cannot always be found." This problem arises because 20 percent of black transplant candidates have markers unique to blacks.[15]

Recent polls indicate that 93 percent of respondents say that they would donate a family member's organs if that person had so requested. And 76 percent said that they would be willing to donate their own organs.[16] Yet the shortage persists. Moreover, it is rather depressing that things have not changed that much during the past two decades.[17] Since one of the major objectives of medicine is to save lives and since many more lives can be saved if more organs are available for transplantation, society seemingly has an obligation to see whether there is a way to secure a greater number of suitable cadaver organs.

What sort of policy should our society adopt for obtaining cadaver organs? At least three possibilities should be examined.[18] To acquire organs from the newly dead, society might adopt a *giving* policy, a *trading* policy, or a policy of *presumed consent*. Let us examine each of these.

As the name implies, the giving policy relies totally on donations. The sole source of cadaver organs for transplantation comes from those people who, before their deaths, have agreed to contribute or whose relatives now agree. The United States has adopted the giving policy. In order to provide some direction and clarity to state laws, the Uniform Anatomical Gift Act was drafted in 1968. This was not a legal statute but rather a model designed by interested citizens to guide the various states. Some version has been adopted by all fifty states. One of the principal purposes of this act was to allow the wishes of deceased persons to donate their organs to stand even if the next of kin were to protest; respecting autonomy was a major goal. The five major provisions of the act are stated here:[19]

1. Person eighteen years or older may donate all or part of their bodies for research or transplantation purposes.
2. Surviving relatives may make a donation if the deceased has left no instructions regarding this matter.
3. If the person has made such a gift, it cannot be revoked by relatives.
4. If there is more than one next of kin, the gift from relatives will not be accepted if any of them has an objection.
5. The gift can be authorized if the person carries a card or if written or verbal communication has been recorded by a relative.

Several comments are in order here. The first clarification concerns provision 5. While organ donor cards are still available, now most states enable people to record their desire to be donors on their driver's license.

Second, there is usually a legal pecking order regarding surviving relatives. Although this might vary from state to state, normally if you are married, your spouse will speak for you regarding organ donations. If you are not married but have adult children, they are next. And if you have neither a spouse nor adult children, then your parents or siblings will speak for you.

Third, although each state has adopted some version of the Uniform Anatomical Gift Act, provision 3 is seldom, if ever, followed. The reality is that even if you have indicated on both your driver's license and an organ donor card your desire to contribute your organs after death, if the person legally authorized to speak for you protests, your organs will not be used. Such a practice, of course, defeats the purpose of enabling you to control what happens to your body after death. There is a practical reason for not opposing the wishes of living relatives, however. Any protests that they make are apt to result in bad publicity for that organ procurement center. Given the shortage of available organs and that in any particular case no usable organs may be available anyway, it simply makes no sense for those charged with obtaining cadaver organs to oppose the wishes of living relatives. From a utilitarian perspective, they are more apt to do their cause harm than good if they act against the wishes of living relatives. Many think that this should change and that the deceased's autonomously expressed wishes should be honored; but for now the reality is otherwise.

Finally, the National Transplant Act of 1984 prohibits the buying or selling of human organs in the United States.[20]

The giving policy, at least as originally conceived, has certain advantages. Most importantly, this policy is designed to respect an individual's right to autonomy. It recognizes that a person's body is his own property and that the owner should control its disposition. In addition, this policy gives people opportunities to perform significant acts of generosity, giving their bodies to help others.

The giving policy poses difficulties, however. First, as already noted, too few people are donating their organs. If most people had religious or moral objections to having parts of their bodies removed after they die, then this would not be a serious objection. It would simply be an indication that many people disapprove of the use of cadaver organs for transplantation, and a society that respects its citizens' autonomy must allow them to refuse. But the evidence suggests that the vast majority of the people in the United States approve of using cadaver organs for transplantation. Given this point and that society has provided a mechanism for people to donate their organs, the shortage is a real problem. Perhaps people are lazy or just not motivated to give. In order to make the giving policy work better, critics say that it will have to be much more aggressive, which is the second objection. Pressure will have to be exerted on people, and in some cases when they are ill and least able to resist.

Finally, a giving policy such as that embodied in the Uniform Anatomical Gift Act has the disadvantage of requiring family approval at the time of death, the time when the family is least likely to provide that approval. Young, healthy persons who have died in an accident or of injuries to the head are among the most suitable donors. Organs from these people are typically far more useful than those from persons who are elderly or have suffered from debilitating diseases. Yet their family members are likely to be in shock and perhaps feel guilty too. In any case, it will be difficult for them to approve of the harvesting of organs from their loved one. The giving policy, then, has not attracted enough donors and does not enable us to secure the organs from the most suitable donors.

Not everyone is ready to abandon the giving policy. Many think that the main problems can be overcome. Proponents of the giving policy believe that it can procure many more organs if only the public is better educated. Many are not aware of the value of organ donation, and others have gross misconceptions about it—for example, that it will cost donor families and that the body of their loved one will be too mutilated to display at a funeral home. An aggressive education campaign using the media, churches, and civic organizations might well do a lot of good.

Already one step has been taken to provide better information. In 1991, so-called "required request" laws went into effect, directing any hospital receiving federal funds to alert family members of seriously ill patients that they have the option of donating organs upon death. Of course, this policy still requires approaching families at a bad time. But it does ensure that they will be made aware of the options. And one suspects that as this practice becomes common, hospital employees charged with this responsibility will become adept at conversing with families in a manner that is sensitive but at the same time persuasive. It is probably too early to determine whether these laws have had desirable effects.

One worry about this practice should be noted. As indicated, polls show that people are more willing to donate the organs of a deceased relative than they are their own. As family members increasingly become the target of organ procurement campaigns, we must wonder whether the autonomy of the newly dead is being violated. If the person did not want to contribute or was hesitant to do so, the consent of the next of kin is tainted.[21]

The trading policy is the second approach that a society might employ for obtaining cadaver organs. Such a policy is based on the idea that people must be provided an incentive to allow their organs to be used when they die. As an inducement, these potential contributors are offered something in return. One obvious possibility is to offer financial compensation. If people sign a document agreeing to contribute their organs upon death, then they will be paid a given amount of money. As another possibility, society could pool all cadaver organs for transplantation and allow only those who have themselves previously agreed to contribute their organs to have access to these organs as a medical resource.[22] In this setup, people would be trading usable organs upon death in exchange for the right to use any available organs that they might need while alive. Each of these versions of the trading policy, however, is open to objections.

The first form of the trading policy would probably be too costly. In order to induce people to contribute their organs, in all likelihood the payment will have to be large. And since the pool of potential contributors must be large (because not everyone's organs will be usable), the total cost will be significant. Some may protest that saving lives is worth considerable cost, saying, "If it saves one life, it is worth it." But this is a cliché that does not really seem to be embraced by most people. Certainly many lives could be saved if the speed limit on interstate highways were reduced to forty miles per hour and enforced strictly. But apparently (judging by behavior) the inconveniences of this policy are too great. In addition, critics say that this version of the trading policy will put most of the burden of contributing organs on the poor. They, after all, will be the ones most motivated to trade for pay.

Finally, the trade-for-pay system seems cumbersome and too easy to abuse. For example, if each state controls its own system and persons who have already been paid move to another state, what happens? In our highly mobile society, this is likely to occur often. And suppose that some who have already been paid claim to have converted to a religion that requires that one be buried intact. This will put policy makers in a difficult position. Either they will have to act against a person's alleged religious beliefs and open themselves to lawsuits from relatives and other members of that religious sect, or they will have to demand repayment of the money already paid (and one suspects that it will be very difficult to recoup these funds in many cases).

The other version of the trading policy is open to different objections. One must admit that something seems initially appealing about making organs for transplantation available only to those who have themselves agreed to contribute their organs. This appeals to a sense of fairness: those who reap the benefits should be willing to bear their fair share of the burdens. But this policy has both practical and moral problems. On the practical side, when must people declare their intentions to contribute? Obviously young children and teenagers must be allowed access to the organs even though they have not agreed to give. But must we demand that a person agree by a specified age, say twenty-one, or else that person is forever ineligible? This seems inappropriate; if a twenty-five-year-old decides to participate, we should welcome her to the pool. But where do we draw the line? If we do not draw the line somewhere, then many people will agree to contribute only when they realize that they need access to the pool, which will defeat the purpose of increasing the pool of *healthy* donors. It is not easy to see how this practical problem can be overcome.

A moral problem is evident too. As a method of distributing a scarce resource, this policy has the potential for great waste. Suppose that at a particular time the only people who both need an available organ for transplantation and are compatible with the potential donor have themselves not yet agreed to contribute their organs. Not allowing one of them to use the organ seems both foolish and immoral, since the alternative is to waste a lifesaving medical resource. This objection about wasting a valuable resource can be overcome if the trade-for-access policy does not exclude persons who have not agreed to donate but instead simply gives priority to those who have agreed to contribute. The Republic of Singapore reportedly adopted such a policy in 1986, with good results.[23]

These criticisms prompt many to dismiss the trading policy as an implausible option. But recently a rather different version of this policy has received serious support.[24] These new suggestions are based on the reality that it is the families of potential contributors who determine whether organs will be procured. So it is family members who need to be provided with incentives. As a result, some have proposed that contributors' families be paid a flat fee—say, $1,000—if they donate the deceased's organs. Another proposal recommends that the contributors' burial fees be paid if organs are procured. One problem with the giving system is that families are reluctant to agree to donation, regardless of whether the newly dead has signed a donor card. A financial reward may overcome this reluctance.

Assuming that one of these versions of the trading policy would significantly increase the supply of available cadaver organs, should it be adopted? There still seem to be problems. Some object that the cost of this system may be great, depending on how much payment must be made to induce relatives to contribute. Some counter, however, that paying donor families may actually be less costly than the current system because if the supply of organs for transplantation is increased, society will save money that it now spends on the treatment of patients awaiting transplants.[25] Another objection is that the vast majority of persons motivated to contribute in this system are likely to be poor. There may be an even more significant problem, however. If families stand to benefit financially from contributing organs of a newly deceased relative, they may be inclined to do this even if the relative had expressly requested that it not be done. We have already noted that the role of the family in the giving policy can result in acting against the potential donor's wishes. But that difficulty may be even greater in this modified version of the trading policy.

This last problem has given rise to a kind of hybrid proposal, one that has features of the giving and trading policies. It operates as a kind of insurance policy. Individuals can agree to donate their organs upon death by signing a contract. The contract designates beneficiaries who will receive a payment if organs are judged medically suitable for transplantation and are taken from the potential contributor. This approach allows individuals to control their own destiny and at the same time provides families with an incentive not to oppose the wishes of the deceased.[26]

Problems may still persist. The system may be quite costly, though for now evidence on this matter is not available. Presumably, in this system we would still allow a family to donate a relative's organs who had not signed the contract, but in that case we would not pay because it would provide families with an incentive to go against the wishes of the deceased. But then one wonders how many such families will contribute. Will they resent the fact that others are being paid?

Let us now examine the third general policy for obtaining cadaver organs for transplantation. It is the policy of presumed consent. A society that adopts this policy salvages any of a person's usable organs upon death unless that person has explicitly requested that this not be done. Several countries are reported to have a policy of routinely salvaging organs from the newly dead, including Austria, Denmark, Finland, France, Greece, Israel, Italy, Norway, Spain, Sweden, and Switzerland.[27] The giving policy puts the burden of proof on those who wish to contribute their organs; they must "opt in" and take steps to indicate their desire to contribute. The policy of presumed consent puts the burden on those who do not want to contribute their organs; they must "opt out" and take positive steps to indicate that they do not want to participate. Organs from minors and other incompetents will not be taken without the consent of the guardian, even in this policy. A society presumably will adopt the policy of presumed consent only if the giving and trading policies are deemed to be inadequate.

The policy of presumed consent has obvious advantages. First, in all likelihood it will greatly increase the supply of available organs. In fact, the only system that could provide more suitable organs would be one that did not allow persons the option of refusing to contribute. Second, such a system can be efficient and not costly. Since organs will not be purchased, the only costs will be in setting up a system so that organs can be procured immediately upon a person's death. And some will argue that this system still respects people's autonomy because it allows them to be buried intact by stating that desire.

Objections have been raised against the policy of presumed consent, however. First, some critics claim that this system puts an unfair burden on patients in hospitals. These people must state any objections they have at a time when they are least able to do so. Second, the policy of routinely salvaging organs from the newly dead will deprive people of the opportunity to exercise generosity.[28] If people voluntarily agree to donate their organs upon death, their actions have a moral quality that they lack if they are forced to contribute. This opportunity to be generous is missing in a society that opts for the policy of presumed consent. The state will seize the organs anyway unless the person has protested; merely not protesting does not seem to be an act of generosity. Third, some worry that if this policy is implemented, then health care professionals will be tempted to hasten a person's death in order to save the life (lives) of a more salvageable patient(s). Health care practitioners may begin to look at dying patients as a potential resource for others, which would affect treatment decisions. And fourth, some think that the policy of presumed consent will be costly and difficult to administer.[29] If the rights of all people to control their bodies are to be respected, society will have to have a centralized registry that can be checked upon a person's death to determine whether he has "opted out." Moreover, this registry will have to be updated continuously, which is likely to be quite costly and cumbersome to administer.

Recently, the policy of presumed consent has been defended against some of these objections.[30] Consider the objection that the policy will put too much pressure on those who are seriously ill because it forces them to register their protests at a time when they are vulnerable. This need not be the case. If the policy of presumed consent is adopted, it will be a public policy of which people are (or should be) aware. People who have religious or moral objections to having organs removed after death will be able to state those objections any time. And certainly if our society were to implement the policy of presumed consent, mechanisms would be readily available for those who chose not to contribute. Indeed, persons who had religious objections would be motivated to move quickly to register them.

With respect to the second objection, defenders of the policy of presumed consent may well grant that it deprives people of one significant opportunity to exercise the virtue of generosity—namely, to donate their organs after death. But as things stand now, in the United States, too few are being generous in this regard. We can admit that it would be better to live in a world in which all of the cadaver organs needed were available because people donated them. However, when an adequate supply of cadaver organs is not being donated, this objection seems weak. Moreover, many other opportunities are available for persons to be generous.

Concerning the third criticism, advocates of the policy of presumed consent can make a simple reply: this objection, if realistic, is applicable to all policies. If health care practitioners might be tempted to see dying patients as potential resources for more salvageable ones, this temptation will exist no matter what policy society adopts. This seems unlikely, however. If a particular health care team knew that a patient of theirs would be the recipient of organs from a dying patient in that same institution, maybe this temptation would exist. But the organs must be distributed to compatible patients, and they will usually be in other institutions, often in other states. In addition, those directly involved in the procurement of organs are not likely to be the primary care givers.

Where does this leave us? Undoubtedly, more lives could be saved if the policy of presumed consent were adopted. Even if required request laws and a national multimedia campaign result in increased donors in the giving system, that result will likely fall short of what the policy of presumed consent could acquire. If the giving policy is to be defended, therefore, it will have to be at a more fundamental level. One might argue, for example, that the policy of presumed consent inappropriately forces people to benefit others. Statutes that require this are usually called *Good Samaritan laws*. One basis for opposing such laws is to maintain that the proper function of the state is to prevent people from harming others. But for a state to compel its citizens to bestow benefits on others is inappropriate. Since the policy of presumed consent would do just that, it should be rejected. By contrast, the giving policy appropriately recognizes that bestowing benefits is an act of charity that must be freely chosen by individuals. Those who share this ideal of a limited state will probably find this defense of the giving policy persuasive.

But this may not be the only ground on which the giving policy can be defended. If educative efforts succeed in increasing the supply of cadaver organs significantly, that may be enough for now. For such a development may make the benefits of organ donation obvious to more people, which may result in even more contributors. It is too early to say whether this optimistic scenario will play out. If it does not, our society will have to consider alternatives. And, indeed, there is some reason to be pessimistic. One recent study suggests that required request policies have not resulted in significant increases in organ procurement.[31] The study indicates that health care professionals are doing a good job of identifying donor-eligible patients and that in most cases families of those patients are approached about donation. In the majority of cases, however, families decline to contribute. Perhaps we should look closer at the hybrid policy mentioned earlier, the one that provides financial incentives to relatives of potential donors, but only of those who have explicitly agreed to contribute while alive. This hybrid policy still respects autonomy while acknowledging the need to provide relatives with incentives..

Another variation on the giving policy advocated recently is called *mandated choice*.[32] This policy would require individuals to state their preferences regarding organ donation when they renew their driver's licenses, file tax forms, or perform some other task required by the state, and then those preferences would have to be honored. This approach would overcome one major obstacle to organ donation: the reluctance of people to contemplate their own deaths before the onset of major illness or injury. Polls indicate that 89 percent of would-be donors have not discussed their wishes with their families.[33] Some may dispute the legitimacy of forcing people to make such a choice. In addition, family members would still have to make decisions regarding donations from children.

Obtaining Renewable Medical Resources

Renewable medical resources are obtained from living human beings, and their loss is temporary. The best-known example of this type of resource is blood. Bone marrow is another example of a renewable medical resource. Blood is obviously a valuable medical resource; often it saves lives. It is a potentially scarce resource for several reasons.[34] First, not everyone can safely donate blood. Some cannot serve as donors because it will adversely affect their own health; others cannot because they would transmit diseases to recipients of their blood. Second, human blood deteriorates. Some parts of blood can be preserved as a useful medical resource for only about three weeks. Third, not only must blood be available, but it must be the right type. A mismatch of types can be lethal. And since some blood types are rare, there is a natural shortage.

What sort of policy should be adopted for obtaining renewable medical resources such as blood? Four possibilities will be discussed here. One policy is the *donorship system*, which is akin to the giving policy explained earlier. In this system, society's entire supply of blood comes from people's voluntary contributions. No incentives are provided.

A second policy for obtaining blood is the *free-market system;* this parallels the trading policy discussed earlier. In such a system, people are paid for contributing blood. Donations, of course, will be accepted, but any contributor who wishes will be paid.

The *taxation system* is a third policy. In this system all of those who are medically suitable will be required to contribute blood. How often each will be required to contribute will depend on how many contributors there are and how much blood is needed. Of course, contributions will not be so frequent as to create a medical hazard for those from whom blood is taken.

A fourth possibility for obtaining blood is the *penalty system*. A society that adopts this policy will obtain at least part of its blood from persons who have been convicted of minor offenses. For example, instead of fining people for exceeding the speed limit, a judge may order them to contribute blood. Judge Irving Goldblatt of Holyoke, Massachusetts, actually issued such an order in 1978, though this is not a general policy in the United States.

How should societies choose among these different systems? What criteria should be appealed to in assessing them? In comparing these four policies, at least the following four criteria should be employed: the cost of the system, the quality of blood obtained by the system, the efficiency of the system, and the moral acceptability of the system. Cost is a simple criterion. If one system can obtain the same quantity of a scarce resource for less money than its competitors, then if other things are equal the less costly system is superior. The quality of blood that each policy is apt to attract is very important. Because many diseases can be transmitted from contributors to recipients through blood, it is important that a policy does not attract so-called "bad blood." An efficient system involves as little waste as possible, which is important because parts of the blood can only be preserved for approximately three weeks. Finally, moral advantages or objections might be associated with the various policies. These may be due either to the inherent nature of the policies or the consequences of adopting them.

Let us begin by using these four criteria to compare the free-market system with the donorship system. Much has been written about this topic.[35] At one time, the free-market system was employed in the United States, and the donorship system was used in Great Britain. Each system had its defenders and critics. Beginning with the criterion of cost, the comparison seems easy. The free-market system is far more expensive. Costs are involved with each system; machinery must be set up for taking in and processing blood. But the free-market system bears an additional cost: contributors are paid. Those defending the free-market system are apt to argue that unless financial incentives are provided, the supply of blood will be inadequate. However, if the donorship system can attract enough donors, it will have an advantage over the free-market system.

SCARCE MEDICAL RESOURCES || **239**

Two examples from the past are illustrative of the problem of "bad blood." Certain forms of hepatitis can be transmitted from carrier contributors to patients who receive their blood. At one time, no test was available that could reliably detect carriers of certain types of hepatitis. A second example is more recent. Until 1985, there was no way to detect the presence of HIV, the virus that causes AIDS, in contributors' blood, and this virus can be passed from carriers to recipients through blood. Any time situations like these arise, the honesty of contributors with respect to their health, medical histories, drug habits, and the like is essential. Recipients' lives will be endangered if contributors are not truthful, especially when answering questions about their medical histories. So it is important to ask what will encourage honesty in this setting. In particular, the motives of likely contributors must be examined (at least in any context where it is possible that a person has a medical problem that can be transmitted to a recipient but cannot be detected by testing the blood).

Consider first the free-market system. Persons who sell their blood apparently need money. This is confirmed by the fact that in the past contributors were paid very little. If people are contributing blood because of a desperate need for money, they will have a strong incentive to conceal any medical problems that might disqualify them from being contributors. Thus, people who had had hepatitis but needed money would be inclined to lie about that fact. And if contributors of blood in the early 1980s had been paid, persons who were HIV-positive and in dire financial straits would be tempted to lie.

In the donorship system, donors' motives appear altruistic; they want to help others. If that is the case, then contributors in the donorship system should be motivated to be truthful in answering questions about their health and medical histories, assuming that they are cognizant of the dangers involved. They will not want recipients to receive their blood if it will have harmful effects.

On this basis, the quality of blood obtained by the donorship system is argued to be superior to that obtained by the free-market system. This point is reinforced by the fact that the incidence of hepatitis is higher among the poor than the general population, and the poor are more likely to sell their blood. If contributors in the donorship system come from all segments of the population, then it will probably attract far less bad blood than the free-market system.

What about the efficiency of the donorship and free-market systems? When the free-market system of the United States was compared with the donorship system as it operated in England and Wales, it was estimated that the American system wasted ten times as much blood as the British system, proportionately. This suggests that the free-market system is less efficient than the donorship system. The crucial question, however, is why the United States' system wasted more blood. To show that the free-market system is inherently less efficient, critics would have to demonstrate that it is more wasteful because it pays for blood, which may be difficult. Some have suggested that the reason the United States' system was more wasteful was that the price it charged for blood did not adequately reflect its scarcity; thus, people were encouraged to use it in a wasteful manner. Others have suggested that at times too many people contributed. Through careless monitoring, more blood was purchased than was needed, thereby causing waste. Whatever the real story is, it is difficult to say that the donorship system is inherently more efficient that the free-market system.

Finally, let us discuss the moral acceptability of these two systems. Are there moral advantages associated with either the donorship system or the free-market policy? Defenders of the donorship system have pointed to two considerations to support the contention that the free-market system is morally inferior to the donorship system. First, they claim that the free-market system exploits the poor. They argue that most of the contributors in a society operating with the free-market system are poor, and many have little prospect of being anything but poor. Some frequent contributors are the temporarily poor, such as graduate students and medical students. Others are those whose economic status is likely more permanent.

Even if this is acknowledged as a fact, however, one might make two different responses to it.[36] Those who criticize the free-market system on moral grounds maintain that people should never take advantage of others because of their social positions. If anything is done, it should be to try to improve those bad conditions. The critics seem to be committed to this position. On the other hand, defenders of the free-market system regard this arrangement as providing the poor with an opportunity to improve their lot, albeit only slightly. Blood is a medical necessity that can be safely obtained from healthy people. If paying contributors for blood enables society to obtain an adequate supply and improves the position of the poor, this situation is the free market at its best. To deprive the poor of this option is paternalistic. Critics of the free-market system lament the fact that in a society that adopts such a policy, the burden of supplying blood is borne largely by the poor. Defenders of the system rejoice at the fact that this provides the poor with an opportunity of improving their position, even if only marginally.

Critics of the free-market system make a second point to show that the donorship system is morally superior. They argue that a purely voluntary system encourages people to behave altruistically, while the free-market system discourages altruism. They claim that experiments show that in situations calling for an altruistic response, people are more inclined to respond altruistically if they have recently witnessed someone else behaving altruistically. The application of this point to policies for obtaining blood is clear. If some people are known to be paid for contributing blood, few will be motivated to give their blood freely; they may even think themselves foolish to do so. But if people see others freely giving blood, they will be more apt to do so themselves. The promotion of altruism is a morally good thing. And if the donorship system promotes altruism better than does the free-market system, then in that regard it is morally preferable. If the factual assumption underlying this objection is correct, this provides an argument not only for adopting the donorship system but also for widely publicizing the fact that people are giving. It may even provide a utilitarian reason for making exaggerated claims about the number of donors while still stressing the need for more!

Since in the United States today almost all whole blood is donated, the British seem to have won the argument. Still, a controversy persists because agencies in the United States still pay contributors for plasma. A process called plasmapheresis is used to separate plasma and red blood cells. The red cells are then reinjected into the contributor. People can contribute plasma more frequently than whole blood without endangering their well-being. In December 1979, the Food and Drug Administration investigated the Community Blood and Plasma Service of Winston-Salem, North Carolina, an agency that buys plasma. Questions were raised about the health of the contributors, with claims that many had been previously rejected because of problems such as alcoholism and drug abuse. It was also contended that the company exploited the poor. A number of those who sold their plasma were allowed to contribute more frequently than is medically advisable. Critics also claimed that those who sold their plasma were not adequately informed of the possible dangers. All of this has reinforced suspicions about a system that pays for any of the blood that it obtains.

The taxation system requires each person medically able to contribute blood periodically. The chief advantage of this system is that it will supply as much blood as any system can safely obtain. How will this system fare when judged by the four criteria used to assess the donorship and free-market systems? Cost is hard to assess. The blood obtained under this system is free. But costs will be involved in setting up the system. A bureaucratic structure will be necessary to ensure that all medically able persons contribute when their turn comes. The taxation system will certainly cost more than the donorship system, but whether these costs will be prohibitive is difficult to say.

Will a taxation system be efficient, or will it waste too much blood? With so many people contributing, the system will have to be set up so that the supply of blood comes in evenly and not all at once; if not, much that is obtained will deteriorate before it can be used. This should prove to be no obstacle, however. Suppose that able people must contribute once a year. Then the system could be arranged so that they donate on their birthday. Such an arrangement would minimize waste.

Because the taxation system requires all medically suitable persons to contribute, one might think that it would attract more bad blood than any other system. This difficulty is acute for any medical problem that can be transmitted through blood but not detected by testing that blood. The problem is most difficult when would-be contributors are dishonest about their medical histories. Are contributors in a taxation system likely to be dishonest? If the taxation system were implemented, contributing blood would probably be regarded by many as a burden. If so, people would be motivated to avoid this burden if possible. For this reason, those who had had medical problems in the past would likely be honest about that. Indeed, suitable donors might lie to try to avoid the burden of giving. We should not be too cavalier about the "bad blood" problem, however, for the AIDS crisis complicates matters. A person can be HIV-positive for at least several months, and perhaps longer, before that state is revealed by a blood test. As a result, contaminated blood can be passed on unknowingly. This condition can happen in the donorship system too, but we might appropriately wonder whether it would happen more in a society that operates with the taxation system.

Finally, what can be said about the moral acceptability of the taxation system? On the positive side, this system distributes the burden of contributing blood as evenly as possible. Certainly it does not exploit the poor. But some will argue that it is inappropriate for the government to force some people to benefit others. And taking a person's blood might be regarded as even worse than taking hours of a person's labor, as is done when people are forced to pay taxes.

A second objection against this policy is reminiscent of one made against taking cadaver organs: a system that forces people to contribute denies them the opportunity to be altruistic and thereby reduces the moral quality of their acts. Whether these moral objections can be answered will not be addressed here.

The penalty system advocates collecting blood instead of a fine from those who are found guilty of misdemeanors and who are medically suitable to contribute. If such a policy were adopted, it would have to serve as a supplement to some other system; it alone could not collect enough blood. In a society using the taxation system, the penalty system would be unnecessary since the taxation system requires that all medically able persons contribute anyway. The question of adopting the penalty system arises, then, only in a society whose principal means of obtaining blood is either the donorship system or the free-market system. There is no reason to believe that the cost of this supplemental system would create any problems. Efficiency too should cause no special problems; the penalty system will be as efficient as the system it supplements.

Would the penalty system be more likely to attract bad blood? Initially, one might think that it would not. There is no reason to believe that persons who have transmittable diseases are more likely to commit misdemeanors than anyone else. The motivations of those who will be contributors must be examined, however. Under the penalty system, contributing blood will be an alternative to paying a fine. Someone who is medically unable to contribute blood must pay the fine. If a very poor person is convicted of exceeding the speed limit, paying a fine may be beyond his means. If so, such a person will be motivated to lie about his medical history if that history is likely to disqualify him as a contributor. So "bad blood" may be a problem in the penalty system.

Whether the penalty system is morally acceptable depends principally on what sort of punishment for crimes is permissible. Is forcing people to contribute blood an appropriate way of having them repay their debts to society? If taking a person's blood is an unacceptable form of punishment, then we must be prepared to explain how this differs in principle from taking days or months of a person's freedom. These issues must be resolved if we are to oppose the penalty system on moral grounds.

This, then, is a brief look at four different policies that society might employ for obtaining renewable medical resources. Clearly, if an adequate supply of the resource in question can be obtained through the donorship system, then that policy should be adopted. If an adequate supply cannot be obtained through voluntary donations, however, then the alternatives must be examined more seriously.

SUMMARY

Some medical resources are in short supply. When that is the case, two broad questions arise. First, how should we allocate these scarce resources? Second, what policy should we adopt for acquiring more of the resources?

Decisions concerning the allocation of scarce medical resources are often a matter of life or death. This chapter has examined two theories on this issue. Each theory allows that only those who are likely to benefit from the receipt of the scarce resource should be a serious candidate. Beyond that point, they disagree radically. Nicholas Rescher's "social worth" theory recommends that deliberate decisions in allocating scarce resources be made. The aim should be to obtain the optimal outcome for society, which is likely to be achieved by giving preference to those who are apt to live longer, who have dependents, who are likely to contribute more to society in the future, and who have contributed more in the past. James Childress rejects such an approach and recommends instead a method in which luck, not deliberate human choice, determines who among medically qualified candidates will receive the resource.

Cadaver organs are one type of scarce medical resource. Three different policies that might be adopted for obtaining cadaver organs were examined: the giving policy, the trading policy, and the policy of presumed consent. Each has advantages and disadvantages. Of the three, the giving policy places the least burden on people and respects the autonomy of individuals; unfortunately, it has not been successful in generating an adequate supply of organs. The policy of presumed consent will provide the greatest supply of cadaver organs but is seen by some as coercive.

Renewable medical resources, such as blood and bone marrow, must be obtained from living human beings. Among the policies that might be adopted for obtaining these resources are the donorship system, the free-market system, the taxation system, and the penalty system. Judging these policies by the criteria of cost, the quality of the resource obtained, efficiency, and moral acceptability, many have concluded that the donorship system is the best. This opinion is probably correct as long as that system can provide an adequate supply of the resource in question.

Suggestions for Further Reading

Caplan, Arthur L. *If I Were a Rich Man Could I Buy a Pancreas?* (Bloomington: Indiana University Press, 1992), Chapters 9–10.

Childress, James F. "Rationing of Medical Treatment." In Warren T. Reich (ed.), *Encyclopedia of Bioethics* (New York: Free Press, 1978), pp. 1414–1419.

Childress, James F. "Who Shall Live When Not All Can Live?" *Soundings*, Vol. 43 (1970), pp. 339–355.

Council on Ethical and Judicial Affairs (of the American Medical Association). "Strategies for Cadaveric Organ Procurement: Mandated Choice and Presumed Consent." *Journal of the American Medical Association*, Vol. 272 (1994), pp. 809–812.

Council on Ethical and Judicial Affairs (of the American Medical Association). "Financial Incentives for Organ Procurement." *Archives of Internal Medicine*, Vol. 155 (1995), pp. 581–589.

Iserson, Kenneth V. *Death to Dust* (Tucson, AZ: Galen, 1994).

Jarvis, Rupert. "Join the Club: A Modest Proposal to Increase the Availability of Donor Organs." *Journal of Medical Ethics*, Vol. 21 (1995), pp. 199–204.

Kilner, John F. *Who Lives? Who Dies?* (New Haven, CT: Yale University Press, (1990).

Lamb, David. *Organ Transplants and Ethics* (New York: Routledge, 1990).

Mathieu, Deborah (ed.). *Organ Substitution Technology: Ethical, Legal, and Public Policy Issues* (Boulder, CO: Westview, 1988).

Munson, Ronald (ed.). *Intervention and Reflection: Basic Issues in Medical Ethics*, 4th ed. (Belmont, CA: Wadsworth, 1992), Chapter 9.

Muyskens, James L. "An Alternative Policy for Obtaining Cadaver Organs for Transplantation." *Philosophy & Public Affairs*, Vol. 8 (1978), pp. 88–99.

Ramsey, Paul. *The Patient as Person* (New Haven, CT: Yale University Press, 1970), pp. 198–215, 239–266.

Rescher, Nicholas. "The Allocation of Exotic Medical Lifesaving Therapy." In Ronald Munson (ed.), *Intervention and Reflection: Basic Issues in Medical Ethics*, 4th ed. (Belmont, CA: Wadsworth, 1992), pp. 538–549.

Siminoff, Laura A., Robert Arnold, Arthur Caplan, Beth Vining, and Deborah Seltzer. "Public Policy Governing Organ and Tissue Procurement in the United States." *Annals of Internal Medicine*, Vol. 123 (1995), pp. 10–17.

Veatch, Robert M. *Case Studies in Medical Ethics* (Cambridge, MA: Harvard University Press, 1977), Chapter 9.

Veatch, Robert M. *Death, Dying, and the Biological Revolution*, rev. ed. (New Haven, CT: Yale University Press, 1989), Chapter 8.

Notes

1. "Moses Cone Study Aims to Slow HIV," *Greensboro News and Record*, May 11, 1993.

2. For a discussion of this case, see Paul Ramsey, *The Patient as Person* (New Haven, CT: Yale University Press, 1970), pp. 242–248.

3. See Ramsey, *The Patient as Person*, p. 246.

4. See Shana Alexander, "They Decide Who Lives, Who Dies," *Life*, November 9, 1962, pp. 102–110, 115–128; and David Sanders and Jesse Dukeminier,

Jr., "Medical Advance and Legal Lag: Hemodialysis and Kidney Transplantation," *U.C.L.A. Law Review*, Vol. 15 (1968). Many of these criticisms are noted by Ramsey, *The Patient as Person*, pp. 246–249.

5. The former claim is made by Alexander, "They Decide Who Lives, Who Dies"; the latter, by Sanders and Dukeminier, "Medical Advance and Legal Lag."

6. Nicholas Rescher, "The Allocation of Exotic Medical Lifesaving Therapy," in Ronald Munson (ed.), *Intervention and Reflection: Basic Issues in Medical Ethics*, 4th ed. (Belmont, CA: Wadsworth, 1992), pp. 538–549.

7. James F. Childress, "Who Shall Live When Not All Can Live?" *Soundings*, Vol. 43 (1970), pp. 339–355; reprinted in Samuel Gorovitz, Ruth Macklin, Arthur Jameton, John O'Connor, and Susan Sherwin (eds.), *Moral Problems in Medicine*, 2d ed. (Upper Saddle River, NJ: Prentice Hall, 1983), pp. 640–649.

8. See Bernard Dickens, "Ethics Committees, Organ Transplantation and Public Policy," *Law, Medicine and Health Care*, Vol. 20 (1992), pp. 300–306.

9. Most of these points are discussed by Ramsey, *The Patient as Person*, pp. 255–259.

10. This case is discussed by Paul A. Freund, "Organ Transplants: Ethical and Legal Problems," in Gorovitz et al. (eds.), *Moral Problems in Medicine*, pp. 637–640.

11. This position is defended by Edmund Cahn, *The Moral Decision* (Bloomington: Indiana University Press, 1955), pp. 61–71. For a critical discussion, see Ramsey, *The Patient as Person*, pp. 259–266.

12. Kenneth V. Iserson, *Death to Dust* (Tucson, AZ: Galen, 1994), pp. 53–55.

13. Arthur L. Caplan, *If I Were a Rich Man Could I Buy a Pancreas?* (Bloomington: Indiana University Press, 1992), pp. 146–147.

14. Since many donors give more than one organ, this figure does not represent the number of organs donated.

15. For the material in this paragraph, see Maria Johnson, "Black Organ Donors Closing the Gap in Transplant Needs," *Greensboro News and Record*, November 11, 1992; Prerna Mona Khanna, "Scarcity of Organs for Transplant," *Wall Street Journal*, September 8, 1992; and "Organ Donations Fail to Increase Despite Donors' Willingness," Associated Press, *Greensboro News and Record*, March 31, 1993.

16. See "Organ Donations Fail to Increase Despite Donors' Willingness." See also Iserson, *Death to Dust*, p. 58.

17. For an account of these developments, see Robert M. Veatch, *Death, Dying, and the Biological Revolution*, rev. ed. (New Haven, CT: Yale University Press, 1989), Chapter 8.

18. These issues are discussed in detail by James L. Muyskens, "An Alternative Policy for Obtaining Cadaver Organs for Transplantation," *Philosophy and Public Affairs*, Vol. 9 (1978), pp. 88–99. Much of my presentation is borrowed from this excellent article.

19. See Veatch, *Death, Dying, and the Biological Revolution*, pp. 213–214. See also Muyskens, "An Alternative Policy for Obtaining Cadaver Organs for Transplantation," pp. 89–90; and Iserson, *Death to Dust*, p. 65.

20. Iserson, *Death to Dust*, p. 78.

21. For a discussion of this point, see Veatch, *Death, Dying, and the Biological Revolution*, pp. 215–216.

22. For a defense of the policy in which access to organs for transplantation is granted *only* to those who have themselves previously agreed to contribute, see Rupert Jarvis, "Join the Club: A Modest Proposal to Increase the Availability of Donor Organs," *Journal of Medical Ethics*, Vol. 21 (1995), pp. 199–204.

23. Iserson, *Death to Dust*, p. 78.

24. For a description of these new suggestions, see Khanna, "Scarcity of Organs for Transplant Sparks a Move to Legalize Financial Incentives."

25. Iserson, *Death to Dust*, p. 78.

26. Council on Ethical and Judicial Affairs (of the American Medical Association), "Financial Incentives for Organ Procurement," *Archives of Internal Medicine*, Vol. 155 (1995), pp. 581–589.

27. See Veatch, *Death, Dying, and the Biological Revolution*, pp. 213, 264 (note 62). It should also be pointed out that in fourteen states in the United States, specific permission to take *eyes* from cadavers is not required; these states have presumed consent laws for this particular tissue. In 1991, 43,000 corneal transplants were performed in the United States, with more than 90 percent of those resulting in restored vision. See Iserson, *Death to Dust*, pp. 72–73.

28. These first two objections are discussed in Ramsey, *The Patient as Person*, p. 210.

29. Caplan, *If I Were a Rich Man Could I Buy a Pancreas?*, p. 152.

30. Some of the points made here are in Muyskens, "An Alternative Policy for Obtaining Cadaver Organs for Transplantation," pp. 94–98. Muyskens refers to what here is called the policy of presumed consent as "the taking policy."

31. Laura A. Siminoff, Robert Arnold, Arthur Caplan, Beth Vining, and Deborah Seltzer, "Public Policy Governing Organ and Tissue Procurement in the United States," *Annals of Internal Medicine*, Vol. 123 (1995), pp. 10–17.

32. Council on Ethical and Judicial Affairs (of the American Medical Association), "Strategies for Cadaveric Organ Procurement: Mandated Choice and Presumed Consent," *Journal of the American Medical Association*, Vol. 272 (1994), pp. 809–812.

33. Iserson, *Death to Dust*, p. 58.

34. Two articles reprinted in Gorovitz et al. (eds.), *Moral Problems in Medicine* have greatly influenced my presentation of this material. They are Richard M. Titmuss, "Why Give to Strangers?" pp. 632–635, and A. J. Culyer, "Letters: Ethics and Economics in Blood Supply," pp. 636–637. See also Peter Singer, "Altruism and Commerce," *Philosophy and Public Affairs*, Vol. 2 (1972), pp. 312–319, and Robert M. Solow, "Blood and Thunder," *Yale Law Journal*, Vol. 80 (1971), pp. 1696–1711.

35. See the articles mentioned in note 34.

36. Here one is reminded of the two positions that might be taken regarding the use of people who volunteer to be experimental subjects only because of the abjectness of their social conditions. See the discussion of the Willowbrook case in Chapter 6, pp. 209–210.

APPENDIX

Codes of Ethics

THE HIPPOCRATIC OATH [1]

I swear by Apollo Physician and Asclepius and Hygieia and Panaceia and all the goddesses, making them my witness, that I will fulfill according to my ability and judgment this oath and this covenant:

To hold him who has taught me this art as equal to my parents and to live my life in partnership with him, and if he is in need of money to give him a share of mine, and to regard his offspring as equal to my brothers in male lineage and to teach them this art—if they desire to learn it—without fee and covenant; to give a share of precepts and oral instruction and all other learning to my sons and to the sons of him who has instructed me and to pupils who have signed the covenant and have taken an oath according to the medical law, but to no one else.

I will apply dietetic measures for the benefit of the sick according to my ability and judgment; I will keep them from harm and injustice.

I will neither give a deadly drug to anybody if asked for it, nor will I make a suggestion to this effect. Similarly I will not give to a woman an abortive remedy. In purity and holiness I will guard my life and my art.

I will not use the knife, not even on sufferers from stone, but will withdraw in favor of such men as are engaged in this work.

Whatever houses I may visit, I will come for the benefit of the sick, remaining free of all intentional injustice, of all mischief and in particular of sexual relations with both female and male persons, be they free or slaves.

What I may see or hear in the course of the treatment or even outside of the treatment in regard to the life of men, which on no account one must spread abroad, I will keep to myself holding such things shameful to be spoken about.

If I fulfil this oath and do not violate it, may it be granted to me to enjoy life and art, being honored with fame among all men for all time to come; if I transgress it and swear falsely, may the opposite of all this be my lot.

FUNDAMENTAL ELEMENTS OF THE PATIENT-PHYSICIAN RELATIONSHIP[2]

The following report of the Council on Ethical and Judicial Affairs was adopted by the AMA House of Delegates on June 26, 1990.

From ancient times, physicians have recognized that the health and well-being of patients depends on a collaborative effort between physician and patient. Patients share with physicians the responsibility for their own health care. The patient-physician relationship is of the greatest benefit to patients when they bring medical problems to the attention of their physicians in a timely fashion, provide information about their medical condition to the best of their ability, and work with their physicians in a mutually respectful alliance. Physicians can best contribute to this alliance by serving as their patients' advocate and by fostering the following rights:

1. The patient has the right to receive information from physicians and to discuss the benefits, risks, and costs of appropriate treatment alternatives. Patients should receive guidance from their physicians as to the optimal course of action. Patients are also entitled to obtain copies or summaries of their medical records, to have their questions answered, to be advised of potential conflicts of interest that their physicians might have, and to receive independent professional opinions.

2. The patient has the right to make decisions regarding the health care that is recommended by his or her physician. Accordingly, patients may accept or refuse any recommended medical treatment.

3. The patient has the right to courtesy, respect, dignity, responsiveness, and timely attention to his or her needs.

4. The patient has the right to confidentiality. The physician should not reveal confidential communications or information without the consent of the patient, unless provided for by law or by the need to protect the welfare of the individual or the public interest.

5. The patient has the right to continuity of health care. The physician has an obligation to cooperate in the coordination of medically indicated care with other health care providers treating the patient. The physician may not discontinue treatment of a patient as long as further treatment is medically indicated, without giving the patient sufficient opportunity to make alternative arrangements for care.

6. The patient has the basic right to have available adequate health care. Physicians, along with the rest of society, should continue to work toward this goal. Fulfillment of this right is dependent on society providing resources so that no patient is deprived of necessary care because of an inability to pay for the care. Physicians should continue their traditional assumption of a part of the responsibility for the medical care of those who cannot afford essential health care.

DECLARATION OF GENEVA[3]

Medical vow adopted by the General Assembly of The World Medical Association at Geneva, Switzerland, September 1948, and amended by the Twenty-Second World Medical Assembly, Sydney, Australia, August 1968.

At the Time of Being Admitted as a Member of the Medical Profession:

I solemnly pledge myself to consecrate my life to the service of humanity.

I will give to my teachers the respect and gratitude which is their due;

I will practice my profession with conscience and dignity;

The health of my patient will be my first consideration;

I will respect the secrets which are confided in me; even after the patient has died.

I will maintain by all the means in my power, the honor and the noble traditions of the medical profession;

My colleagues will be my brothers;

I will not permit considerations of religion, nationality, race, party politics or social standing to intervene between my duty and my patient.

I will maintain the utmost respect for human life, from the time of conception; even under threat, I will not use my medical knowledge contrary to the laws of humanity.

PATIENT'S BILL OF RIGHTS[4]

The American Hospital Association presents a patient's Bill of Rights with the expectation that observance of these rights will contribute to more effective patient care and greater satisfaction for the patient, his physician, and the hospital organization. Further, the Association presents these rights in the expectation that they will be supported by the hospital on behalf of its patients, as an integral part of the healing process. It is recognized that a personal relationship between the physician and the patient is essential for the provision of proper medical care. The traditional physician-patient relationship takes on a new dimension when care is rendered within an organizational structure. Legal precedent has established that the institution itself also has a responsibility to the patient. It is in recognition of these factors that these rights are affirmed.

1. The patient has the right to considerate and respectful care.

2. The patient has the right to obtain from his physician complete current information concerning his diagnosis, treatment, and prognosis in terms the patient can be reasonably expected to understand. When it is not medically advisable to give such information to the patient, the information should be made available to an appropriate person in his behalf. He has the right to know by name, the physician responsible for coordinating his care.

3. The patient has the right to receive from his physician information necessary to give informed consent prior to the start of any procedure and/or treatment. Except in emergencies, such information for informed consent, should include but not necessarily be limited to the specific procedure and/or treatment, the medically significant risks involved, and the probable duration of incapacitation. Where medically significant alternatives for care or treatment exist, or when the patient requests information concerning medical alternatives, the patient has the right to such information. The patient also has the right to know the name of the person responsible for the procedures and/or treatment.

4. The patient has the right to refuse treatment to the extent permitted by law, and to be informed of the medical consequences of his action.

5. The patient has the right to every consideration of his privacy concerning his own medical care program. Case discussion, consultation, examination, and treatment are confidential and should be conducted

discreetly. Those not directly involved in his care must have the permission of the patient to be present.

6. The patient has the right to expect that all communications and records pertaining to his care should be treated as confidential.

7. The patient has the right to expect that within its capacity a hospital must make reasonable response to the request of a patient for services. The hospital must provide evaluation, services and/or referral as indicated by the urgency of the case. When medically permissible a patient may be transferred to another facility only after he has received complete information and explanation concerning the needs for and alternatives to such a transfer. The institution to which the patient is to be transferred must first have accepted the patient for transfer.

8. The patient has the right to obtain information as to any relationship of his hospital to other health care and educational institutions insofar as his care is concerned. The patient has the right to obtain information as to the existence of any professional relationships among individuals, by name, who are treating him.

9. The patient has the right to be advised if the hospital proposes to engage in or perform human experimentation affecting his care or treatment. The patient as the right to refuse to participate in such research projects.

10. The patient has the right to expect reasonable continuity of care. He has the right to know in advance what appointment times and physicians are available and where. The patient has the right to expect that the hospital will provide a mechanism whereby he is informed by his physician or a delegate of the physician of the patients continuing health care requirements following discharge.

11. The patient has the right to examine and receive an explanation of his bill regardless of source of payment.

12. The patient has the right to know what hospital rules and regulations apply to his conduct as a patient.

No catalogue of rights can guarantee for the patient the kind of treatment he has a right to expect. A hospital has many functions to perform, including the prevention and treatment of disease, the education of both health professionals and patients, and the conduct of clinical research. All these activities must be conducted with an overriding concern for the patient, and, above all, the recognition of his dignity as a human being. Success in achieving this recognition assures success in the defense of the rights of the patient.

THE NUREMBERG CODE[5]

1. The voluntary consent of the human subject is *absolutely* essential. This means that the person involved should have legal capacity to give consent; should be so situated as to be able to exercise free power of choice, without the intervention of any element of force, fraud, deceit, duress, overreaching, or other ulterior form of constraint or coercion; and should have sufficient knowledge and comprehension of the elements of the subject matter involved as to enable him to make an understanding and enlightened decision. This latter element requires that before the acceptance of an affirmative decision by the experimental subject there should be made known to him the nature, duration, and purpose of the experiment; the method and means by which it is to be conducted; all inconveniences and hazards reasonably to be expected; and the effects upon his health or person which may possibly come from his participation in the experiment.

The duty and responsibility for ascertaining the quality of the consent rests upon each individual who initiates, directs, or engages in the experiment. It is a personal duty and responsibility which may not be delegated to another with impunity.

2. The experiment should be such as to yield fruitful results for the good of society, unprocurable by other methods or means of study, and not random and unnecessary in nature.

3. The experiment should be so designed and based on the results of animal experimentation and a knowledge of the natural history of the disease or other problem under study that the anticipated results will justify the performance of the experiment.

4. The experiment should be so conducted as to avoid all unnecessary physical and mental suffering and injury.

5. No experiment should be conducted where there is an *a priori* reason to believe that death or disabling injury will occur; except, perhaps, in those experiments where the experimental physicians also serve as subjects.

6. The degree of risk to be taken should never exceed that determined by the humanitarian importance of the problem to be solved by the experiment.

7. Proper preparations should be made and adequate facilities provided to protect the experimental subject against even remote possibilities of injury, disability, or death.

8. The experiment should be conducted only by scientifically qualified persons. The highest degree of skill and care should be required through all stages of the experiment of those who conduct or engage in the experiment.

9. During the course of the experiment the human subject should be at liberty to bring the experiment to an end if he has reached the physical or mental state where continuation of the experiment seems to him to be impossible.

10. During the course of the experiment the scientist in charge must be prepared to terminate the experiment at any stage, if he has probable cause to believe, in the exercise of the good faith, superior skill, and careful judgment required of him that a continuation of the experiment is likely to result in injury, disability, or death to the experimental subject.

DECLARATION OF HELSINKI[6]

Recommendations guiding medical doctors in biomedical research involving human subjects, adopted by the Eighteenth World Medical Assembly, Helsinki, Finland, 1964, and revised by the Nineteenth World Medical Assembly, Tokyo, Japan, 1975.

Introduction

It is the mission of the medical doctor to safeguard the health of the people. His or her knowledge and conscience are dedicated to the fulfillment of this mission.

The Declaration of Geneva of the World Medical Association binds the doctor with the words, "The health of my patient will be my first consideration," and the International Code of Medical Ethics declares that, "Any act or advice which could weaken physical or mental resistance of a human being may be used only in his interest."

The purpose of biomedical research involving human subjects must be to improve diagnostic, therapeutic and prophylactic procedures and the understanding of the aetiology and pathogenesis of disease.

In current medical practice most diagnostic, therapeutic or prophylactic procedures involve hazards. This applies *a fortiori* to biomedical research.

Medical progress is based on research which ultimately must rest in part on experimentation involving human subjects.

In the field of biomedical research a fundamental distinction must be recognized between medical research in which the aim is essentially diagnostic or therapeutic for a patient, and medical research, the essential object of which is purely scientific and without direct diagnostic or therapeutic value to the person subjected to the research.

Special caution must be exercised in the conduct of research which may affect the environment, and the welfare of animals used for research must be respected.

Because it is essential that the results of laboratory experiments be applied to human beings to further scientific knowledge and to help suffering humanity, The World Medical Association has prepared the following recommendations as a guide to every doctor in biomedical research involving human subjects. They should be kept under review in the future. It must be stressed that the standards as drafted are only a guide to physicians all over the world. Doctors are not relieved from criminal, civil and ethical responsibilities under the laws of their own countries.

I. Basic Principles

1. Biomedical research involving human subjects must conform to generally accepted scientific principles and should be based on adequately performed laboratory and animal experimentation and on a thorough knowledge of the scientific literature.

2. The design and performance of each experimental procedure involving human subjects should be clearly formulated in an experimental protocol which should be transmitted to a specially appointed independent committee for consideration, comment and guidance.

3. Biomedical research involving human subjects should be conducted only by scientifically qualified persons and under the supervision of a clinically competent medical person. The responsibility for the human subject must always rest with a medically qualified person and never rest on the subject of the research, even though the subject has given his or her consent.

4. Biomedical research involving human subjects cannot legitimately be carried out unless the importance of the objective is in proportion to the inherent risk to the subject.

5. Every biomedical research project involving human subjects should be preceded by careful assessment of predictable risks in com-

parison with foreseeable benefits to the subject or to others. Concern for the interests of the subject must always prevail over the interest of science and society.

6. The right of the research subject to safeguard his or her integrity must always be respected. Every precaution should be taken to respect the privacy of the subject and to minimize the impact of the study on the subject's physical and mental integrity and on the personality of the subject.

7. Doctors should abstain from engaging in research projects involving human subjects unless they are satisfied that the hazards involved are believed to be predictable. Doctors should cease any investigation if the hazards are found to outweigh the potential benefits.

8. In publication of the results of his or her research, the doctor is obliged to preserve the accuracy of the results. Reports of experimentation not in accordance with the principles laid down in this Declaration should not be accepted for publication.

9. In any research on human beings, each potential subject must be adequately informed of the aims, methods, anticipated benefits and potential hazards of the study and the discomfort it may entail. He or she should be informed that he or she is at liberty to abstain from participation in the study and that he or she is free to withdraw his or her consent to participation at any time. The doctor should then obtain the subject's freely-given informed consent, preferably in writing.

10. When obtaining informed consent for the research project, the doctor should be particularly cautious if the subject is in a dependent relationship to him or her or may consent under duress. In that case the informed consent should be obtained by a doctor who is now engaged in the investigation and who is completely independent of this official relationship.

11. In case of legal incompetence, informed consent should be obtained from the legal guardian in accordance with national legislation. Where physical or mental incapacity makes it impossible to obtain informed consent, or when the subject is a minor, permission from the responsible relative replaces that of the subject in accordance with national legislation.

12. The research protocol should always contain a statement of the ethical considerations involved and should indicate that the principles enunciated in the present Declaration are complied with.

II. Medical Research Combined with Professional Care (Clinical Research)

1. In the treatment of the sick person, the doctor must be free to use a new diagnostic and therapeutic measure, if in his or her judgment it offers hope of saving life, reestablishing health or alleviating suffering.

2. The potential benefits, hazards and discomfort of a new method should be weighed against the advantages of the best current diagnostic and therapeutic methods.

3. In any medical study, every patient—including those of a control group, if any—should be assured of the best proven diagnostic and therapeutic method.

4. The refusal of the patient to participate in a study must never interfere with the doctor-patient relationship.

5. If the doctor considers it essential not to obtain informed consent, the specific reasons for this proposal should be stated in the experimental protocol for transmission to the independent committee (1, 2).

6. The doctor can combine medical research with professional care, the objective being the acquisition of new medical knowledge, only to the extent that medical research is justified by its potential diagnostic or therapeutic value for the patient.

III. Non-Therapeutic Biomedical Research Involving Human Subjects (Non-Clinical Biomedical Research)

1. In the purely scientific application of medical research carried out on a human being, it is the duty of the doctor to remain the protector of the life and health of that person on whom biomedical research is being carried out.

2. The subjects should be volunteers—either healthy persons or patients for whom the experimental design is not related to the patient's illness.

3. The investigator or the investigating team should discontinue the research if in his/her or their judgment it may, if continued, be harmful to the individual.

4. In research on man, the interest of science and society should never take precedence over considerations related to the well-being of the subject.

AMERICAN MEDICAL ASSOCIATION ETHICAL GUIDELINES FOR CLINICAL INVESTIGATION [7]

The following guidelines are intended to aid physicians in fulfilling their ethical responsibilities when they engage in the clinical investigation of new drugs and procedures.

1. A physician may participate in clinical investigation only to the extent that those activities are a part of a systematic program competently designed, under accepted standards of scientific research, to produce data which are scientifically valid and significant.

2. In conducting clinical investigation, the investigator should demonstrate the same concern and caution for the welfare, safety, and comfort of the person involved as is required of a physician who is furnishing medical care to a patient independent of any clinical investigation.

3. Minors or mentally incompetent persons may be used as subjects in clinical investigation only if:

    A. The nature of the investigation is such that mentally competent adults would not be suitable subjects.

    B. Consent, in writing, is given by a legally authorized representative of the subject under circumstances in which informed and prudent adults would reasonably be expected to volunteer themselves or their children as subjects.

4. In clinical investigation primarily for treatment—

    A. The physician must recognize that the physician-patient relationship exists and that professional judgment and skill must be exercised in the best interest of the patient.

    B. Voluntary written consent must be obtained from the patient, or from the patient's legally authorized representative if the patient lacks the capacity to consent, following: (a) disclosure that the physician intends to use an investigational drug or experimental procedure, (b) a reasonable explanation of the nature of the drug or procedure to be used, risks to be expected, and possible therapeutic benefits, (c) an offer to answer any inquiries concerning the drug or procedure, and (d) a disclosure of alternative drugs or procedures that may be available. Physicians should be completely objective in discussing the details of the drug or procedure to be employed, the pain and discomfort that may be anticipated, known risks and possible hazards, the quality of life to be expected, and particularly the alternatives. Especially, physicians should not use persuasion to obtain consent which otherwise might not be forthcoming, nor should expectations be encouraged beyond those which the circumstances reasonably and realistically justify.

    i. In exceptional circumstances, where the experimental treatment is the only potential treatment for the patient and full disclosure of information concerning the nature of the drug or experimental procedure or risks would pose such a serious psychological threat of detriment to the patient as to be medically contraindicated, such information may be withheld from the patient. In these circumstances, such information should be disclosed to a responsible relative or friend of the patient where possible.

    ii. Ordinarily, consent should be in writing, except where the physician deems it necessary to rely upon consent in other than written form because of the physical or emotional state of the patient.

    iii. Where emergency treatment is necessary, the patient is incapable of giving consent, and no one is available who has authority to act on the patient's behalf, consent for standard therapy only is assumed.

5. In clinical investigation primarily for the accumulation of scientific knowledge—

    A. Adequate safeguards must be provided for the welfare, safety and comfort of the subject. It is fundamental social policy that the advancement of scientific knowledge must always be secondary to primary concern for the individual.

    B. Consent, in writing, should be obtained from the subject, or from a legally authorized representative if the subject lacks the capacity to consent, following: (a) disclosure of the fact that an investigational drug or procedure is to be used, (b) a reasonable explanation of the nature of the procedure to be used and risks to be expected, and (c) an offer to answer any inquiries concerning the drug or procedure.

6. No person may be used as a subject in clinical investigation against his or her will.

7. The overuse of institutionalized persons in research is an unfair distribution of research risks. Participation is coercive and not voluntary if the participant is subjected to powerful incentives and persuasion.

8. The ultimate responsibility for the ethical conduct of science resides within the institution (academic, industrial, public, or private) which conducts scientific research and with the individual scientist. Research institutions should assure that rigorous scientific standards are upheld by each of their faculty, staff, and students and should extend these standards to all reports, publications, and databases produced by the institution. All medical schools and biomedical research institutions should implement guidelines for a review process for dealing with allegations of fraud. These guidelines should ensure that (a) the process used to resolve allegations of fraud does not damage science, (b) all parties are treated fairly and justly with a sensitivity to reputations and vulnerabilities, (c) the highest degree of confidentiality is maintained, (d) the integrity of the process is maintained by an avoidance of real or apparent conflicts of interest, (e) resolution of charges is expeditious, (f) accurate and detailed documentation is kept throughout the process, and (g) responsibilities to all involved individuals, the public, research sponsors, the scientific literature, and the scientific community is met after resolution of charges. Academic institutions must be capable of, and committed to, implementing effective procedures for examining allegations of scientific fraud. No system of external monitoring should replace the efforts of an institution to set its own standards which fulfill its responsibility for the proper conduct of science and the training of scientists.

9. With the approval of the patient or the patient's lawful representative, physicians should cooperate with the press and media to ensure that medical news concerning the progress of clinical investigation or the patient's condition is available more promptly and more accurately than would be possible without their assistance. On the other hand, the Council does not approve of practices designed to create fanfare, sensationalism to attract media attention, and unwarranted expressions of optimism because of short-term progress, even though longer range prognosis is known from the beginning to be precarious. With the approval of the patient or the patient's family, the Council, however, encourages the objective disclosure to the press and media of pertinent information. If at all possible, the identity of the patient should remain confidential if the patient or the patient's family so desires. The situation should not be used for the commercial ends of participating physicians or the institutions involved.

Notes

1. Reprinted with permission of the publisher from Owsei Temkin and C. Lilian Temkin (eds.), *Ancient Medicine: Selected Papers of Ludwig Edelstein* (Baltimore: Johns Hopkins University Press, 1967), p. 6.

2. Reprinted with the permission of the American Medical Association. Published in *Journal of the American Medical Association*, Vol. 264 (Dec. 26, 1990), p. 3133. Copyright 1990, American Medical Association.

3. Reprinted with the permission of the World Medical Association.

4. Reprinted with the permission of the American Hospital Association.

5. Reprinted from *Trials of War Criminals before the Nuremberg Military Tribunals* (Washington, DC: U.S. Government Printing Office, 1948).

6. Reprinted with permission from the World Medical Association.

7. Reprinted with permission from the American Medical Association. Source: *Code of Medical Ethics: Current Opinions with Annotations.* Copyright 1994, American Medical Association.

INDEX